WHAT THE BIBLE SAYS ABOUT HEALTHY LIVING

THREE BIBLICAL PRINCIPLES THAT WILL CHANGE YOUR DIET AND IMPROVE YOUR HEALTH

REX RUSSELL MD

3559

Fleming H. Revell

A Division of Baker Book House Co
Grand Rapids, Michigan 49516

Worldwide coedition organized and
produced by
Angus Hudson Ltd,
Concorde House, Grenville Place,
Mill Hill, London NW7 3SA, England
Tel: +44 181 959 3668
Fax +44 181 959 3678

Printed in Singapore

Contents

Foreword

I first met Rex Russell in Vermont in the fall. The colors of autumn were painting the leaves into a beautiful landscape as we bicycled mile after mile along narrow roads in that beautiful state. Rex told me of his desire to write this book, and I encouraged him to do so. I am glad he did because he has clearly shown us a way to live healthier lives.

Rex is one of the funniest people I know. As you begin reading this book, I encourage you to turn to chapter 7 and read his account of his initial introduction into radiology during his first year of residency. This will give you some understanding of the kind of person Rex is. He has used his good humor, his medical expertise and his knowledge of Scripture to help us learn what can enable us to have good health. He has used his own personal health problem, diabetes, to show us the benefit healthy living can be to all of us. It is not a theoretical proposition to him, nor should it be to us.

Rex has used his deep trust in God and scriptural insights to show how the One who made us knows best how we will function. His emphasis reminds me of my Ford pickup truck. The people who made it provided an owner's manual. They know how they made it, and, therefore, know best how it works. If I follow their instructions, it will run better and last longer.

Rex has clearly shown this truth in his book. God made us, He knows how we will function best and be the healthiest. If we will follow His guidelines, we are more likely to experience His best for us—physically, emotionally and spiritually.

Rex's book is a thorough evaluation of food and drink and its powerful effect on human health. Rex is honest when he admits his stubbornness in making changes in his diet. I am sure each of us can identify with that. My wife and I began making changes in our diets several years ago. I resisted some of those changes strenuously. What I think you will find, as we did, and as Rex so clearly points out, is that as you begin eating a healthier diet you will enjoy that food more. You will also enjoy the improved health that accompanies it.

It would seem that to follow Rex's guidelines would produce a constricted life. Let me encourage you, however, that by doing what he says, the good health that results will allow you to have a freer life in the future— a life freer of illness, tiredness and depression than the life you will live if you don't follow the guidelines he, and I believe God, has planned for us.

God is real and is a God who really did create us. His love is shown by the way He has given us clear direction in the way He meant for us to live in His Word, the Bible.

I encourage you to not just read what Rex has written, but also to put it into practice. He has done us all a great service by adding more light to the path of life and health.

Joe S. McIlhaney, Jr., M.D.
Medical Institute for Sexual Health
Austin, Texas

Check Your Health IQ

Based on your present view of health, you might enjoy taking a quiz about foods and other aspects of health. You can check your answers as you learn more about the divine design for health as described in this book. If you enjoy treasure hunting, you can search the text for answers. If you like to cut to the chase, see appendix 1.

Mark items that are good for your health with a +.
Mark items that are bad for your health with a −.
Mark 0 if it doesn't matter.
Mark the worst eight items for your health with an * (eight points).
Each correct answer = 1 point.

1. fiber	23. pork
2. nuts	24. homogenized milk
3. whole-grain cereals	25. soft drinks
4. sunlight	26. same-spouse sex
5. swordfish	27. juice
6. marriage	28. smoking
7. "Type A" personality	29. cover fat on meat
8. "Type B" personality	30. anger
9. bitterness	31. blond hair
10. olive oil	32. sunglasses
11. butter	33. shellfish
12. margarine	34. prayer
13. safe sex (condom)	35. alcohol
14. wine	36. fasting
15. rest	37. forgiveness
16. same-gender sex	38. breast feeding
17. live fruits	39. large-mouth bass
18. avocados	40. catfish
19. sweating from labor	41. smiling
20. sprouts	42. promiscuity
21. live vegetables	43. hot dogs
22. beef	44. divorce

Introduction

My family and I were just not well.

I had known for some 25 years that I was diabetic. Still, for much of my life I was able to participate in sports and otherwise lead a fairly normal life.

Now, however, in 1976, the disease was gaining ground. I also suffered a host of related ailments, including chronic abscesses, arthritis, swelling in my legs and deterioration of my arteries, eyesight and kidneys.

My children were having their own health problems, such as infections, dental abscesses and cavities, and hyperactivity, while other relatives and friends had "hit the wall" with various diseases.

What could I do?

Because I'm a doctor, I searched for medical answers with many physicians. One convinced me that my diet needed more vitamins and minerals. So I began taking about 50 pills a day. I was still ill, and exhausted, but I continued to test such measures and to study the many claims of various scientists and nutritionists. Instead of health and clarity, I only experienced continued illness and confusion.

One evening in desperation I pulled a Bible off the shelf. I happened to come across Psalm 139:14, where the psalmist praises God because "I am fearfully and wonderfully made." Immediately I looked up in anger and said, "If we are so wonderfully made, why am I so sick? God, why didn't You give us a way to be healthy?"

My heavenly answer came in the form of a quiet question in my mind. *Rex*, the Questioner said, *have you really read my Instruction Book?*

Of course I held a Bible on my lap, but I was skeptical that what I might find inside its pages would help. How could a book written between 2,000 and 6,000 years ago possibly have any relevant health information? I knew that in primitive times such as those the best research promoted treating splinters with worm's blood and donkey's dung. I doubted that any ordinances in Scripture could offer any help for modern man.

I was also a little afraid. Even if the Bible were to point me to some answers, would they be taken as ridiculous by other physicians? Would what Scripture had to say move me toward rejecting my faith? I knew that God's reputation rested on His laws. How could any of the some 632 commandments in Deuteronomy, plus other laws scattered throughout Scripture, possibly reinforce my faith, or help in my world, or help me?

Yet I decided to read God's Word for what it might have to say about my plight. I prayed for wisdom from Him alone, because I had not been helped by human ideas about health.

Sure enough, this study brought to me exciting new understanding and insights. The pages of Scripture sprang to life for me.

I began to take seriously the fact that God promised good health to the Jewish people:

> If you listen carefully to the voice of the Lord your God and do what is right in his eyes, if you pay attention to his commands and keep all his decrees, I will not bring on you any of the diseases I brought on the Egyptians, for I am the Lord, who heals you (Exod. 15:26).

Gradually, my wife, Judy, and I began to realize that God's laws in the Old Testament were intended to *bless* His people. This *blessing* was not just a spiritual blessing; it was a holistic blessing, including the Jewish people's health and social structure. Indeed, this is what the Hebrew word *shalom* means: peace, welfare, blessing in all aspects of life. Specifically, the laws God gave His people were both a method God used to teach His people obedience and a way to spare them from many easily preventable illnesses and problems.

Several months later I did some self-examination. I hadn't had an abscess in months. The boils had disappeared, and my health had improved in other ways. This general improvement inspired me to redouble my efforts to discover and apply any principles of health God had for me in His Word.

I began taking about 50 pills a day, but I was still ill and exhausted.

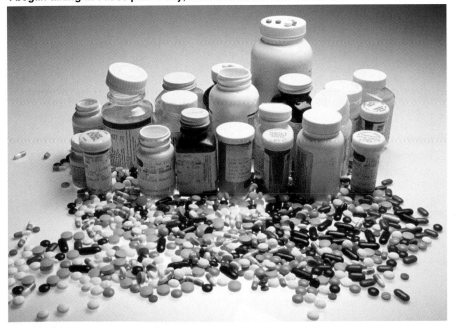

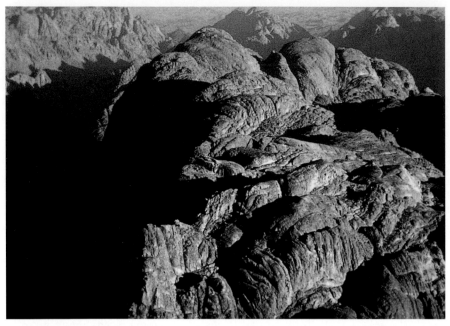

After the Exodus, God promised the Israelites would not suffer the diseases of Egypt.

As I thought about what was happening to me, and why, I wondered about other believers—Jews and Christians—who had far greater Bible knowledge than I had. Why had they ignored this teaching about good health? Was I becoming a fanatic?

During a four-year period of study, the different pieces of the puzzle of health began to fit together. Gradually I came to understand that God gave His laws to protect people, and that astounding measures of health are available to those who obey these laws, whether they are believers or not. I organized what I had learned around three principles I want to share with you in this book.

By following these laws, I have not had one carbuncle (abscess) or any arthritis in the last 18 years. What a change! Before applying these laws, the retina in my eyes had deteriorated to the point that I had to have laser therapy. My retinal surgeon scheduled my appointments every three months to monitor any changes. Now I have 20/20 vision, and my appointments are scheduled every year or two. My doctor, who has a large practice, claims that I've done better than any of her other diabetic patients.

These changes in my health came from personal application of the principles in this book. I have greatly benefited from them, but they are not a cure-all—although I believe they will

"help all." I'm healthier because I try to follow God's principles for healthy living, but I will still face disease. I still have insulin-dependent diabetes. The complications of my disease, however, have been reversed and/or delayed. I am a healthy person.

Neither are these principles another kind of "faith healing." Although many people have studied these principles and obediently applied them, experiencing miraculous results, my own faith was limited. Yet God was true to fulfill His laws in my life. His divine design works.

This book has several purposes. First, I will supply information from both the Bible and medical research about disease prevention. It is reassuring to know that great protection is available to those who will follow God's design for healthy living. Unfortunately, many waste precious resources on unnecessary health expenses.

Some who will read this book lack a personal relationship with the God of the universe. Even so, by following the principles of His Word, they can benefit from His design for healthy living.

I also want this book to help Christians who are sick. The Bible is also a great resource for the recovery of health. Through faith and the power of the Holy Spirit, believers will be able to follow these biblical principles.

As you read through this information, you can quietly apply the Divine Design by yourself, with your family or with a few friends.

So here is an invitation for you to begin your own personal journey to healthier living through the knowledge and application of God's design. In the seventh century before Christ, Hosea, the prophet to the kingdom of Judah, uttered this doleful lament:

My people are destroyed from lack of knowledge (Hos. 4:6).

When Hosea preached this, he was not just speaking to his own historical situation. He was laying out a principle similar to the law of cause and effect. Much like our own generation, Hosea's generation had faithlessly broken the covenant with God (see v. 1), brazenly transgressed the Ten Commandments (see v. 2), thoughtlessly polluted the land with sin (see v. 3) and stubbornly followed after priests who ignored God's laws (see vv. 4,5). Having rejected the knowledge of God, the priests exchanged the glory of God for something disgraceful (see vv. 6-9). Hosea understood and communicated the consequences of ignoring God's law—destruction and death.

I believe that this principle is true in the area of healthful living: If we decide to pay attention to God's design, health and blessing will follow, and God will be glorified in our lives. If we decide to ignore God's design, the consequences can be dire indeed.

In the pages that follow, we will examine commandments, parables and illustrations given by our Designer to help us live healthier, more fruitful lives. As you decide to follow the Designer's commands, He will be glorified in your life.

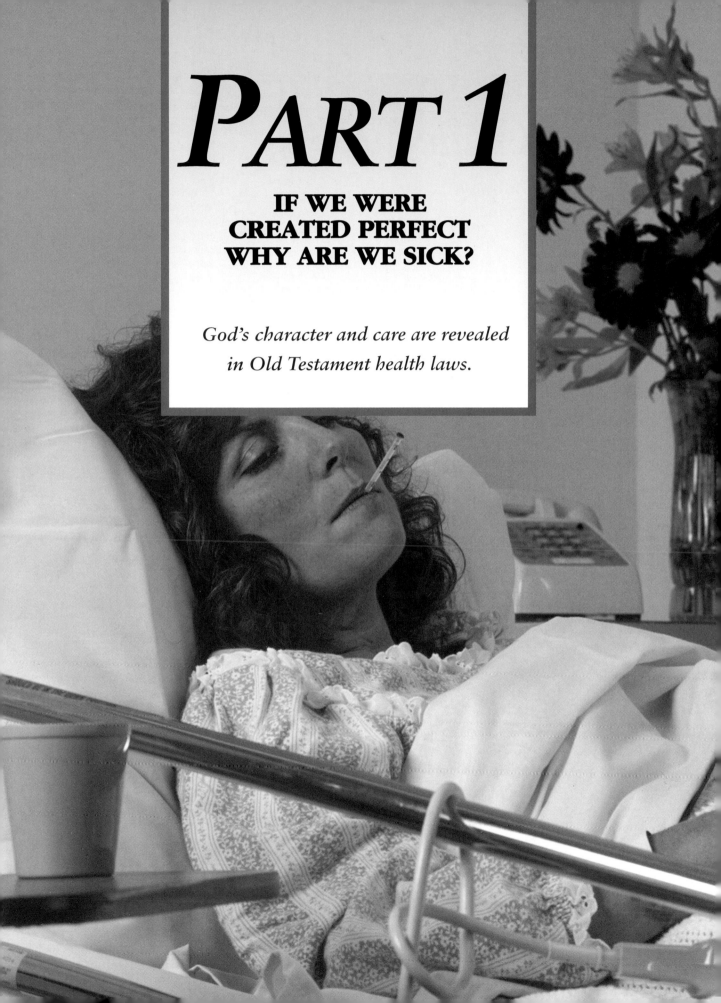

PART 1

IF WE WERE CREATED PERFECT WHY ARE WE SICK?

God's character and care are revealed in Old Testament health laws.

1. Eating Right in a World Gone Wrong

Wouldn't you like to discover a way to regain something of the health God intended for His people?

The hospitals in Vienna, Austria, had a problem. New mothers were dying at a rate of one in six! At the time—in the mid-1800s—physicians who had just examined the recent dead would enter the wards and examine the expectant mothers without washing their hands. Sadly, these doctors were unknowingly spreading bacteria and disease—and death.[1]

This tragedy could have been avoided if the physicians of the day had known and followed the principle God had laid down thousands of years earlier, as recorded in Numbers 19:11:

"Whoever touches the dead body of anyone will be unclean for seven days."

God offered no explanation of this law. Had the physicians in Vienna simply obeyed it, however, hundreds of lives could have been spared.

One Viennese physician, Dr. Ignaz Semmelweiss, searched for a solution to the problem. He required his staff to wash their hands in a bowl of water before examining any patients on his ward. They didn't scrub their hands with soap, as doctors and nurses do today, but only rinsed them.

The death rate in Dr. Semmelweiss's ward dropped to 1 in 84.

As happens with many who develop new ideas, this good doctor wasn't an immediate hero. Instead, he was fiercely attacked for his claims, and faced ridicule and attack from the medical community. Eventually his battle cost him his practice and his sanity.

And, women continued to die until more doctors discovered, through science, the truth of God's Word.

When All Else Fails, Try Reading Directions

Diseases fill our daily lives—everything from the common cold to cancer and high blood pressure. Yet the early pages of Genesis tell of a perfect world designed by a benevolent Designer. What happened?

Early in my studies of the Scriptures, I sought to answer this basic question about illness.

Considering all the sickness and disease we experience today, could it be that we have not listened carefully enough to the voice of the Lord as related in Exodus 15:26?

"If you listen carefully to the voice of the Lord your God and do what is right in his eyes, if you pay attention to his commands and keep all his decrees, I will not bring on you any of the diseases I brought on the Egyptians, for I am the Lord, who heals you."

Just like the doctors in nineteenth-century Vienna (and elsewhere), we have not paid attention to God's instructions regarding healthful living. This is one reason we get sick.

Did you notice that the women who

died in the Viennese hospitals were not necessarily guilty of specific sins? It was their caregivers who did not follow God's law regarding cleanliness. This contributes to a second reason we fall ill: We live in a fallen world. The earth, our home, just hasn't worked as well as it did when God created it, as recorded in Genesis 1. The sad fact is that Genesis 3 happened—we fell, and the earth fell with us, producing all sorts of harmful influences that were not in God's original, grand design.

But the Lord immediately set about instituting His plan of redemption. Eventually it would culminate in God's sending His Son and the blood of Jesus being shed as a sacrifice for our sins. Yet even prior to that "new creation," God gave His people a law to show them their need.

That is the law referred to in Exodus 15. Those commands include dozens of ways to live—morally, spiritually and in good health. The law promised that God's people would suffer "none of these diseases" if they could and would follow His way.

The Perfection of God's Design

As you know, many people in the medical community are not trained to accept the notion that an intelligent Creator designed and created a perfect world. Yet today there has arisen an exciting movement among many doctors and other scientists to reexamine this position. An experience I had in 1967 during my internship at the University of Kentucky illustrates why.

My first surgical case was a newborn male who was scheduled to be circumcised. After finishing the operation, I carefully bandaged the wound. Four hours later, I checked the patient and discovered that the bandage was soaked with blood.

We administered vitamin K to help clot the blood, but a slight bleeding persisted for several days before it completely stopped. A specialist checked the boy and found no evidence of hemophilia. No harm was done, but an infant had begun life

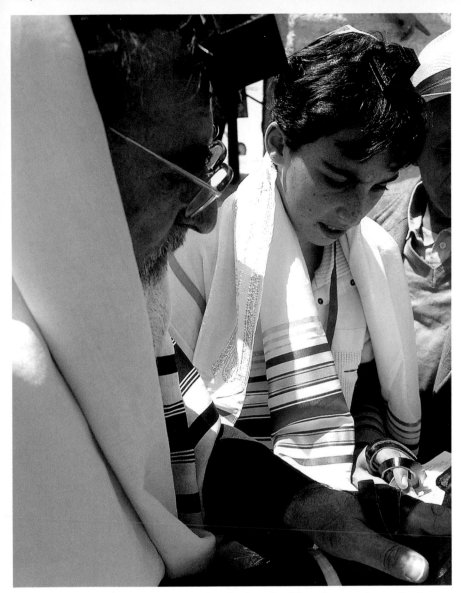

A Jewish boy's barmitzah. Since Abraham's time, Jewish males are circumcised.

circumcision because it teaches a spiritual lesson. Under the Old Covenant, circumcision symbolized the passing from an unclean state (being outside the people of God) to a clean state (being numbered among His people). God told His elect servant Abraham, "It will be the sign of the covenant between me and you" (Gen. 17:11).

When the gospel branched out to Gentiles, this outward sign was no longer required of non-Jewish believers (see Acts 15:1-29; also 1 Cor. 7:18,19). Circumcision, however, remained as a symbol of putting away the old, unclean disposition to sin and accepting the citizenship God gives us among His people (see Rom. 2: 28,29).

The ongoing value of literal circumcision is shown by medical research; it proves that circumcised males have a lower incidence of infections and carcinoma of the penis.[2] Also, the female partners of uncircumcised males have more infections, which in turn result in a higher incidence of cancer of the cervix.

Obeying God's laws leads to health.

A Word About His Word

Before we go any further, let me say a couple of things. My heart for this book is to help you discover a better way of living—what I believe to be God's design for health. And though my intent is not to throw a lot of biblical terminology at you, it's important that we set a firm foundation for our discussion. So let's take a couple of pages and explore how God's views about food are found in both the Old and New Testaments. By exploring these issues, we can better understand how to live healthier lives today—and how God has provided a way for us to achieve better health.

What Value Is Old Testament Law to the Christian?

For many years I believed that the first five books of the Bible (the law of Moses, or the Mosaic law) were only for the Jews. When I would read them, I would skip rapidly over the

with an unnecessary risk.

Why?

It is routine procedure to circumcise babies during the first three days of their lives. The body's natural supply of the blood-clotting vitamin K, however, is not yet present. Research has now shown that this clotting factor in infants is at its lowest level on days two through five. Vitamin K begins to develop in the intestine as the infant nurses. After five to seven days of breast-feeding, infants have built up enough vitamin K to allow blood clotting to withstand circumcision.

Genesis 17:12 says, "For the generations to come every male among you who is eight days old must be circumcised." When we are obedient to this command, the risk during circumcision greatly decreases. As it is, enough

complications occur with early circumcision so that some physicians aren't recommending the procedure at all.

Some scientists assume that the foreskin of the penis was an evolutionary development to protect males before they learned to wear clothing. I believe the foreskin was designed for man's protection as he strolled through the Garden of Eden. But after the Fall, things changed. Clothing was then necessary to protect Adam's sensitive genital area.

Negatively, the foreskin provided a moist, warm area that was an ideal place for harmful bacteria to grow. Because God, the Designer, loves His creation, He was concerned about proper hygiene and gave the commandment to be circumcised.

We can also see the importance of

laws God gave concerning diet, health and disease. After all, doesn't Paul say "we have been released from the law" (Rom. 7:6)?

Kosher Laws

To answer this crucial question, let's draw the distinction between *kosher* laws and Old Testament Mosaic law. *Kosher* laws, observed today by Orthodox Jewish communities, use Old Testament laws as a starting point, but go far beyond the Old Testament in scope and detail. These extra regulations do not come from the Bible, but from Jewish oral tradition, the sayings of the rabbis. These were written down in the *Talmud* between the second and fifth centuries after Christ.[3] Let me be clear: I am not advocating that Christians embrace and follow *kosher* laws, or other aspects of Jewish talmudic tradition.

In addition, according to both the Old and New Testaments, no one has ever been justified before God by observing the Old Testament law (see Gal. 2:16; 5:6; cf. Gen. 15:6). Rather, justification comes by grace through faith in the promise of God (innocent blood must be shed), demonstrated in Jesus Christ and His atoning blood on the cross (see Eph. 2:8,9; Heb. 9:23—10:18). In the same way as we begin our spiritual lives through faith, we continue and finish by faith (see Gal. 3:2,3).

Therefore, observing Old Testament ceremonial or dietary laws or secondary Jewish traditions have absolutely no effect on whether we are ceremonially or spiritually "clean" or "unclean" (see 1 Cor. 8:8). We can clearly see this in the teaching of Jesus Christ and the early New Testament church.

Validity of the Law

Jesus Christ Himself, as did the Old Testament prophets, validated the Law—He did not come "to abolish the Law or the Prophets; . . . but to fulfill them" (see Matt. 5:17). Nevertheless, through His example He overturned the mistaken popular idea that following the entire law of Moses as interpreted by Jewish traditions made a person right with God.[4]

For example, Jesus explicitly con-tradicted rabbinical teaching in Mark 7:1-23. The rabbis assumed that ritual or spiritual defilement came from physical contact with unclean things, such as eating unclean foods. To the Pharisees, and to the disciples, ceremonial impurity was clearly sin. But Jesus taught that the source of spiritual defilement came from within: all His examples of sin in this passage are moral failures, not ceremonial ones. By "declaring all foods clean," I do not believe Jesus was saying any food people happen to eat would henceforth be healthful; rather, He was saying that one's heart attitude toward God is the essential thing.

The whole point of the writer of the book of Hebrews is that the ritual law in all its dimensions—from sacrifices to dietary laws—was merely "a matter of food and drink and various ceremonial washings—external regulations applying until the time of the new order" (Heb. 9:10), anticipating the good things that were coming in Christ for all peoples, both Jews and non-Jews (see Heb. 9:10; 10:1).

The Apostle Paul's Preaching

The pivotal story in the New Testament of how the gospel spread from the mainly Jewish early church to non-Jews (Gentiles) through Peter further underscores the point that Old Testament ceremonial law was fulfilled in Christ.[5]

This episode correlates with the decision of the Jerusalem Council in Acts 15. The Council decided, applying the teaching of Jesus and the preaching of Paul, that Gentiles did not have to follow the entire Mosaic law to attain salvation. The Council decided that Gentiles needed only to avoid foods that would be offensive to religious Jews who believed in Jesus but still followed the Mosaic law (see Acts 15:28,29). Now it was possible for the gospel to rapidly spread among non-Jewish peoples.

Like Jesus and the Jerusalem council, Paul affirmed the abiding rel-

Kosher matzohs—Jewish unleavened bread.

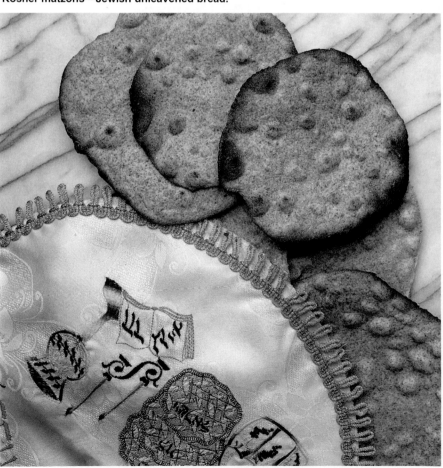

evance of the Old Testament. Like Jesus, Paul boiled down the law to its most essential ingredients (see Matt. 22:37-39; compare with Rom. 13:8-10). In keeping with the New Covenant brought about in Christ, however, Paul taught that the Old Testament categories of clean and unclean no longer have spiritual significance—it was possible to disagree on subjects such as Sabbath practices and circumcision and still be true to the essential gospel message (see Rom. 14:1-18; cf. 1 Cor. 10:23-31; Gal. 5:1-23; Col. 2:16; 1 Tim. 4:4).[6]

We can see that both the theology and the story of the emerging church speaks with one voice: The Church does not negate the Old Testament Law, but fulfills the Old Testament Law in its entirety by faith in Christ through the power and guidance of the Holy Spirit (see Rom. 3:31; 8:3,4).

The Old Testament law is good (see Rom. 7:12; 1 Tim. 1:8). It points to God's glorious, loving, merciful character. The law created a special identity for God's people; it was a means for testing the obedience of His people; and it set Israel apart from the surrounding nations.

As we read the New Testament, however, we see that it does not support the Jewish idea that righteousness and adherence to kosher ceremonial law are related. The law cannot bring us spiritual life (see Rom. 8:3). Only the perfect Messiah who was sacrificed for our sins can do that.

I wholeheartedly agree with the apostle Paul. Just as being circumcised, or not being circumcised, does not have any spiritual value (see 1 Cor. 7:19; Gal. 5:1-23)—so also eating the meat of unclean animals, or not eating the meat of unclean animals, does not have any spiritual value (see 1 Cor. 10:23-31). I believe that no food is spiritually unclean in itself (see Rom. 14:14); however, I believe that eating unclean meat and not being circumcised can result in health problems, many of them serious or even deadly.

Glorify God for His Design

I am urging you, therefore, to take another look at these laws, not for the spiritual purposes of salvation or

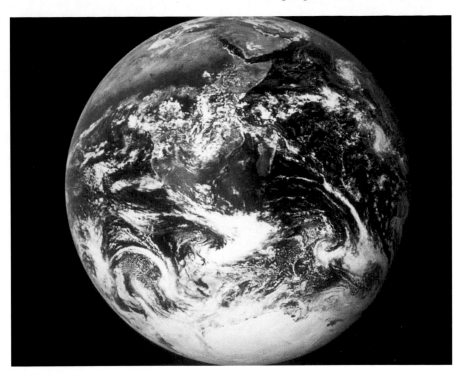

The earth from space. "The universe is the incarnation of a divine intelligence."

sanctification, not to get you to follow Jewish *kosher* laws, or for the purpose of ceremonial purity. Rather, I am urging you to look at these laws *for the purpose of glorifying God through acknowledging His desire and design for our health.*

As Christians, we know that this life on earth is not all there is (see Mark 8:34,35; John 14:1,2; 1 Cor. 6:13), that our days are in God's hands (see Ps. 139:16) and that in the final analysis death will not be victor over us (see 1 Cor. 15:51-55).

We also know that the Lord has given us two great gifts: the gift of life, and the gift of eternal life. He wants us to enjoy what He has created, and to give glory and honor to Him. "The earth is the Lord's, and everything in it" (Ps. 24:1). He wants us to wisely use the good gifts He has given us to seek the profit of others, that they might also come to know the great gift of salvation in Christ that we enjoy (see 1 Cor. 10:31-33).

As the apostle Paul said, "Do you not know that your body is a temple of the Holy Spirit, who is in you, whom you have received from God? You are not your own; you were bought at a price. Therefore honor God with your body" (1 Cor. 6: 19,20).

Therefore, for those who decide to observe health principles derived from Old Testament Mosaic law, the reason for following these principles might be the desire to take care of what God has given you physically, thus glorifying your Creator with your health. For the unconvinced or nonbeliever, the reasons for following these principles could be to test the Law to see if our Creator inspired the Bible. A simpler reason for following these principles may be just because they will improve your health.

Some of God's principles for health were laid down long before Moses arrived on the scene. Circumcision was practiced as early as Abraham's day. Even earlier, God had instructed Noah to take seven of every "clean" animal into the ark, and only one pair of animals that were "unclean." The point is that God has been concerned about our health from the Creation, not just since Moses gave the law. Because He created us, it makes sense that He should know best what makes us healthy!

Science and God

Florence Nightingale, the famous nurse of the last century, wrote in her manuscript *Suggestions for Thought,* "The universe is the incarnation of a divine intelligence that regulates all things through law." For Nightingale, the laws of science were the "thoughts of God." She practiced this philosophy in the field during the Crimean War. Although untrained as a nurse, she used the skills gained through applying her philosophy to become the health consultant to many nations, including the United States; and she is credited with developing the field of nursing.[7]

God's laws work. The laws of science are consistent with the laws of Scripture. They are irrefutable. There are wise and unwise choices in the area of health just as there are in other areas of our lives.

The Prohibition of Blood

In Genesis 7, the Bible first makes the distinction between "clean" and "unclean" animals. In preparation for the great flood, God told Noah:

Take with you seven of every kind of clean animal, a male and its mate, and two of every kind of unclean animal, a male and its mate (v. 2).

After the flood, however, God told Noah that the blood of even *clean animals* was forbidden:

You must not eat meat that has its lifeblood still in it (Gen. 9:4; cf. Lev. 3:17; 7:26,27; 19:26; Deut. 12:16-24; 1 Sam. 14:32-34).

Why did God forbid the consumption of blood? A possible theological answer is that the blood that courses through the veins of animals is an apparent symbol for life. Another answer is that in the sacrificial law, animal blood was provided by God for the atonement of human sin (see Lev. 17:11). Therefore, respect for life, for God the giver of life and the awful penalty for sin are probably reflected in this prohibition. A theological answer, however, does not exhaust the possible explanations.

Scientists have long known that blood carries infections and toxins that circulate in an animal's body. If people eat animal blood, they are needlessly exposed to these infections and toxins.

The Three Principles

Principle I:
Eat only substances God created for food. Avoid what is not designed for food.

Principle II:
As much as possible, eat foods as they were created—before they are changed or converted into something humans think might be better.

Principle III:
Avoid food addictions. Don't let any food or drink become your god.

In Africa, some tribes require the consumption of large amounts of blood in coming-of-age religious ceremonies. Among such tribes, chronic diseases normally associated with the elderly are much more common, and life spans are significantly reduced.

When God commanded that the Israelites abstain from blood, it was not just an arbitrary law; in effect God was sparing the Israelites the plagues and lowered life expectancy that come from eating contaminated blood.

Clean and Unclean

"You must distinguish between the holy and the common, between the unclean and the clean" (Lev. 10:10).

In the law-making period of Israel's history, God was building and solidifying Israel into its particular identity. The distinction between "clean" and "unclean" became more sharply drawn. God wanted to preserve His people for his own purposes—to teach them to separate themselves from idolatry and to trust and believe in Him alone. His reputation depended on the validity of the Law.

"Clean" meant separated *for* God; "unclean" meant separated *from* God. The word "clean" was associated with purity, holiness and being set apart for God, and acting in an ethically righteous way; "unclean" became associated with death, putrefaction, lewdness and demons (see Lev. 11—15; Zech. 13:2; cf. Lev. 19:4; Ps. 106:37-39; Ezek. 22:3).

The laws of purity operated in many areas of life. People who contracted infectious skin diseases such as leprosy became unclean if they had open wounds (see Lev. 13:17,44). God wanted the Israelites to separate themselves from the pagan, idolatrous rituals and beliefs of the surrounding peoples.[8] In the New Testament era, the apostle Paul also warned against the dangers of idolatry.[9]

In the struggle to establish a people and a name for Himself, God gave His people laws that distinguished between clean and unclean on at least three important and overlapping levels. (1) The laws of cleanness and uncleanness had a spiritual level, establishing the one true God as head over all and ousting all rivals. (2) The laws had an ethical level, teaching the Israelites obedience and the holiness of God. As we shall see, however, these two aspects do not completely exhaust the possible explanations. As we look at modern science and nutrition, we will find that (3) there is an amazing overlap between God's original laws of clean and unclean and solid hygienic principles.[10]

Three Important Rules

My study of the Scriptures, my study of medicine and the application of these areas in my life have led me to three core goals or principles that I believe God has imparted to us to live healthier lives. These principles form the foundation of this chapter, and the foundation of this book, for that matter. I call these guidelines simply "The Three Principles."

If you will memorize these three simple principles, a multitude of otherwise confusing decisions about health and diet can be simplified. And

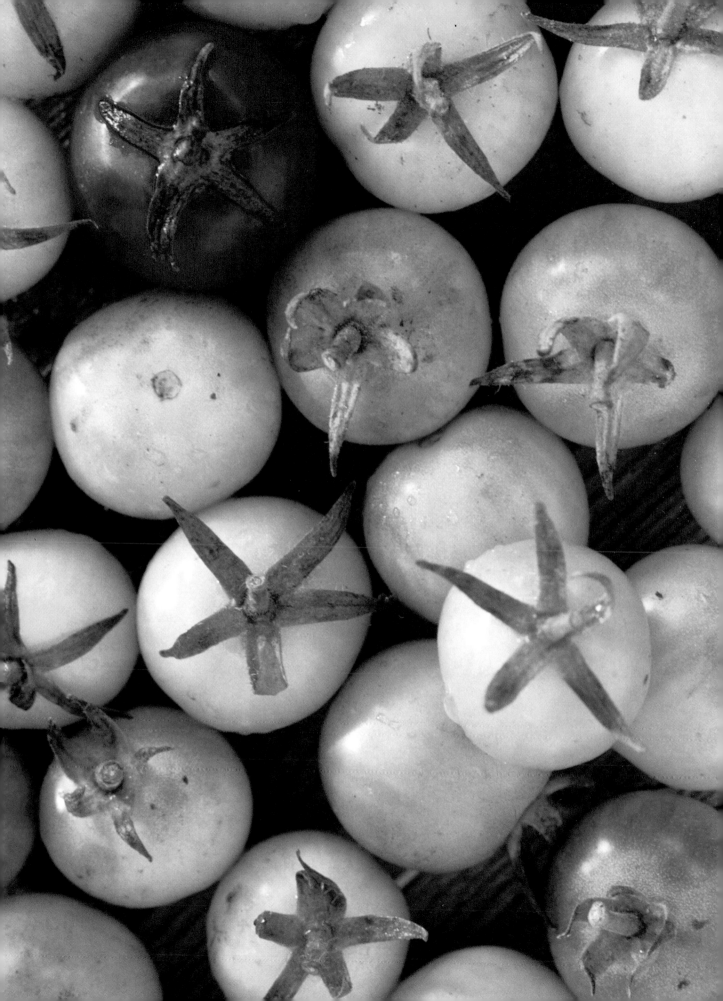

you'll be healthier for it! They are displayed in the panel on p. 14.

Let's examine each of these principles more closely.

Principle I:

EAT ONLY SUBSTANCES CREATED FOR FOOD

A Simply Divine Diet

In the very first chapter of the Bible, God said to humans:

"I give you every seed-bearing plant on the face of the whole earth and every tree that has fruit with seed in it. They will be yours for food" (Gen. 1:29).

Recall that this gift of food was given by God before the Fall of man as recorded in Genesis 3. Not until after the Fall did some plants that had been a part of a perfect creation begin to reflect the sinful nature of humans, for God said even the ground would be cursed (see Gen. 3:17).

Consider the lives of the men and women after the Fall. Adam lived for 930 years in a world filled with the plants and fruits given to him by a loving God. Then after the Fall, and after the Flood, the life expectancy had decreased to the point that Shem, son of Noah, lived "only" 500 years.

Some scientists believe that a great change occurred in the earth's atmosphere and climate after the Flood, which resulted in progressive deterioration of the human life span. Some 1,300 years later, Moses lived only 120 years—and He followed the Law very carefully. Apparently he died in good health (see Deut. 34:7); perhaps our own life span would be similar if we followed the same dietary principles.

Many specialists in aging believe that we have the potential to live, in good health, for about 120 years, too. What happened to shorten our average life expectancy? Can we can make an educated guess by comparing those early people in Scripture with people in our own times? Despite the fact that the United States has the world's best medical facilities, the average life span has only recently increased to 74 years. Did the ancient

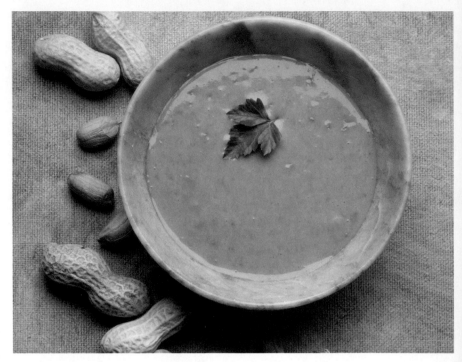

A simple diet of nuts, grains, vegetables and legumes aids healthy living.

psalmist have an insight that applies here?

We are consumed by thine anger, and by thy wrath are we troubled. Thou hast set our iniquities before thee, our secret sins in the light of thy countenance. For all our days are passed away in thy wrath: we spend our years as a tale that is told. The days of our years are threescore years and ten; and if by reason of strength they be fourscore years, yet is their strength labour and sorrow; for it is soon cut off, and we fly away (Ps. 90:7-10, KJV).

Scripture and medical research agree that modern lifestyles lived without reference to God's laws and design shorten life and hasten death.

It has been reported that in the early twentieth century, a people in the Himalayas called the Hunzas had an average life span of 90 years, and often over 120 years. When a medical team led by Dr. Robert McGarrison studied the Hunzas in the 1940s, the physicians did not find a single case of cancer, ulcers, appendicitis or colitis. Heart disease and hypertension were unknown among them. The medical experts also found that the Hunza people ate nuts, grains, vegetables, fruits and legumes. The team could only conclude that the Hunzas' life

expectancy was based on clean water and exercise—and to their adherence to a diet very much like the one described in Genesis 1:29.[11]

In 1949, the Hunzas were incorporated into Pakistan, and their life span has since been shortened because of changes in diet.

Divinely Forbidden Fat

Another illustration of the first principle comes from the book of Leviticus, where God said to Moses:

"Say to the Israelites: Do not eat any of the fat of cattle, sheep or goats" (7:23).

From medical research, we now understand that fat is a tissue in which the body stores energy. When a meal is missed, the body breaks down fat and uses the fat as fuel for energy. Unfortunately, animal fat is also a storage place for toxins and parasites. These toxins are found in the fat of all the animals we eat. Examples include DDT, insecticides, herbicides, antibiotics, hormones and various other chemicals the animals have ingested, breathed or touched.

In 1979, a hormone called DES (diethylstilbestrol) was removed from the market because researchers learned that this substance caused cancer in the vagina and cervix in

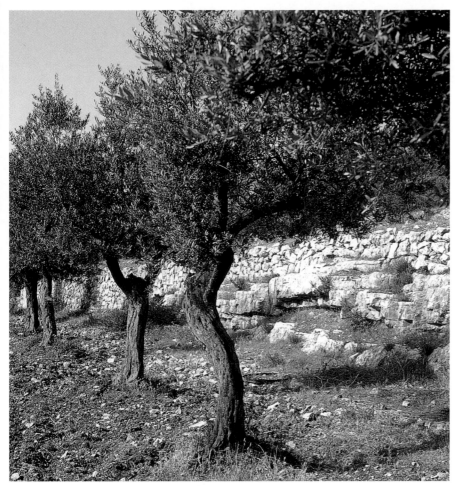

Olive trees cultivated on the Mount of Olives, Jerusalem, Israel.

Bible, olive oil and olive trees are important and a symbol of blessing (see Deut. 7:13; Judg. 9:8-13). Used in cooking and in other ways, olive oil was a valuable commodity for the Israelites. At the time I found this verse in Isaiah 25, however, modern caregivers were saying olive oil was bad for us because it wasn't polyunsaturated.

Then researchers began to note that the Greek people, who consumed large amounts of olive oil, had an extremely low incidence of hardening of the arteries.[13] Further research has shown that olive oil is digested like complex carbohydrates and has healthful fatty acids, which is actually a windfall for health—particularly for a vascular disease such as hardening of the arteries.[14]

Once again, I had to be thankful for a God who knows our makeup so intimately that He provided just the right kind of fat to His people so many hundreds of years ago.

The original sin in Eden involved diet: Adam and Eve ate the forbidden fruit, which was what they wanted instead of what God allowed (see Gen. 3:6). We should remember the punishment for their rebellion:

"Cursed is the ground because of you; through painful toil you will eat of it all the days of your life. It will produce thorns and thistles for you, and you will eat the plants of the field. By the sweat of your brow you will eat your food (Gen. 3:17-19).

Like the original couple, all have rebelled against God (see Rom. 3:23) and lusted after things that aren't good for us—including certain kinds of food. It shouldn't surprise us that what we consume often "consumes" us."

daughters of women who had received the drug to prevent miscarriage. They found that the stockyards throughout the United States injected beef cattle with large amounts of DES because it enabled the animals to gain weight rapidly. And sure enough, the hormone was stored in the animals' fat tissue.

Scientists have also discovered other hormones added to food that produce cancer, and many of these hormones are found in highest concentration in the fat that covers meats.[12]

Hard fat (i.e., fat that is firmest at room temperature and is most saturated) is the most toxic fat for the human body. The increased consumption of hard fats in our day has been accompanied by increased vascular disease, cancers of the breast, colon and prostate, along with many other chronic diseases.

Several years ago I asked a professor of animal husbandry at Oklahoma State, "What animals have the hardest fat?"

Without hesitation the professor replied, "That's easy. The hardest fats are found in cows (oxen), sheep, and goats."

As for me, I sense God's protective hand and a divine design in Leviticus 7:23, where He exclusively lists these three animals.

Is All Fat Bad?

Some people have labeled all fat as harmful. That might be an easy conclusion if we're going only by the information from some caregivers. The Bible doesn't say that all fat is bad. For example, Isaiah prophesied:

In this mountain shall the Lord of hosts make unto all people a feast of fat things (Isa. 25:6, KJV).

When I first read this verse, I thought, *God, you've made a mistake! You shouldn't feed people fat!* Then I dug a little deeper into the passage, and discovered that the best translation for the word "fat" here is liquid oils, including olive oil. In the

---

Principle II:

EAT FOODS AS THEY WERE CREATED

Proverbs 14:12 says:

There is a way that seems right to a man, but in the end it leads to death.

The spiritual truth this proverb

states is that our attempts to be god, to do things our own way, or to earn righteousness by good deeds all lead to spiritual death. The passage also yields a secondary practical truth that provides a good warning against humans' incessant presumption that we can somehow improve on God's design.

In our consumptive and pleasure-seeking culture, we often concoct additives, chemicals and processed foods that take us away from our Creator's excellent design for nutrition.

An Addition That Subtracts

Take the example of how we have tampered with one of our most basic foods—bread. Deuteronomy 32:12-14 lists various substances God has given His people for food. One of the items is "kidneys of wheat" *(KJV)*, which are really the germ layers in a kernel of grain, shaped like a kidney.

This germ layer is so rich with nutrients that, like many rich substances, it spoils quickly in ordinary circumstances. The baking industry, however, has removed more than 20 vitamins and minerals from wheat in its attempt to increase the storage life of bread and prevent spoilage.

The operation was a success, but it wasn't healthy. Our bread now has extended storage life. Because the germ layer in the wheat grain has been removed, bacteria and molds that would spoil the bread can't live on it—and neither can we. These lost nutrients and enzymes are the God-given balance to the kernel; they allow us to thrive, and to digest it properly.

Principle III:

DON'T LET ANY FOOD OR DRINK BECOME YOUR GOD

The third principle is derived from the first commandment:

You shall have no other gods before me (Exod. 20:3).

God has given us good food to eat. Anything good, however, can be made bad by misuse or by allowing it to consume our attention—a place God reserves for Himself.

We commonly use the term "addiction" to describe this difficulty. Researchers have thoroughly documented the chronic effects of addiction to chemicals in substances such as alcohol, drugs and tobacco.

People can also become addicted to foods. Common examples of this are dependencies on caffeine, fat, sugar and salt.

We can also overdo and become addicted to foods God gave for our use. In Deuteronomy 32:13-14, God discusses several foods He has provided for us. Then in verse 15 He charges:

Jeshurun grew fat and kicked; filled with food, he became heavy and sleek. He abandoned the God who made him and rejected the Rock his Savior.

The word "Jeshurun" means "the upright one," and refers to God's people, Israel. God's own people had forsaken Him, substituting for Him an overabundance of food that made them sluggish from gluttony. They were "hooked on food." Both acute and chronic conditions can result from any kind of overconsumption.

Addicts have chronic health problems in every system of their bodies. For example, the alcoholic may have brain atrophy, severe psychic disorders, heart disease, liver disease, bowel disease, joint problems and muscle wasting, along with vague aches, pains and fatigue.

Virtually every organ system is affected when people make alcohol their "god." One whole medical specialty—orthomolecular medicine—is dedicated to studying the chronic illnesses that result from multiple food abuses and/or addictions. These physicians treat chronic diseases that seem to have no causes other than sensitivities or food abuse.

Fasting to Break Addictions

One way to protect ourselves from becoming "hooked," even on otherwise good foods, is to follow God's admonition to spend frequent times with Him alone, without food (see chapter 5).

Fasting is a very effective way of freeing ourselves from preoccupation with our physical wants and desires in order to concentrate on our relationship with God.

A good physical explanation of the benefits of fasting is that during this time of allowing our bodies to rest, the enzyme systems replenish themselves to their proper balance. For

Researchers have documented the effects of addiction to chemicals in alcohol.

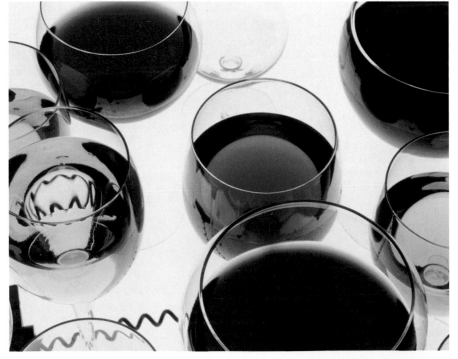

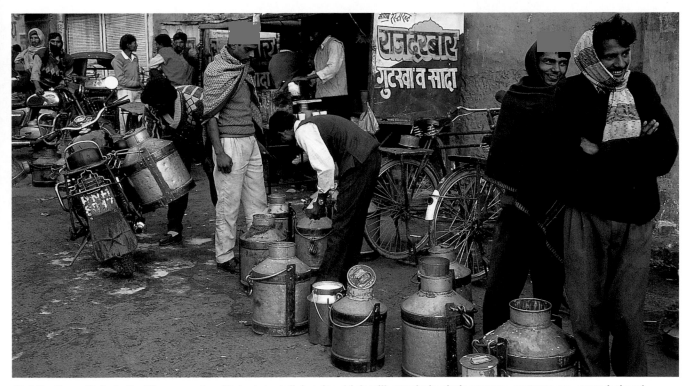

Distributing milk in India. When people with lactate deficiencies drink milk regularly, their enzyme systems are overwhelmed.

instance, people who have lactase deficiencies can usually tolerate milk on an infrequent basis, but when they consume milk products regularly their enzyme systems are overwhelmed. Symptoms such as headaches, irritability, abdominal discomfort and arthritis may soon develop.

In the Bible the activities of fasting include fasting in mourning (see 2 Sam. 1:12; 12:21-23); for seeking God's face (see Jon. 3:5); for obtaining answers to prayer (see Ps. 35:13); for deliverance from enemies and oppressors (see Ezra 8:21,23; Esther 4:16; Ps. 69:10; 109:24); for getting closer to God (see Luke 2:37); for putting ourselves into a position where we can hear from His Word more clearly (see 1 Cor. 7:5); for blanketing a particular decision or problem with prayer (see Dan. 6:18); and for asking God to intervene in our lives for revival and missions (see Acts 13:2,3). The Bible also credits victory in spiritual warfare to fasting (see Matt. 17:21). Clearly, the primary benefits of fasting are spiritual.

When we consider the spiritual benefits of fasting, we may discern a fundamental desire of God that we be free from everything that compromises who God has created us to be. This would include food addictions. As Isaiah said:

Is not this the kind of fasting I have chosen: . . . to set the oppressed free and break EVERY YOKE? (58:6, emphasis mine).

Addicts cannot be considered "free from every yoke" mentally, emotionally and spiritually. When we become physically dependent upon any substance, even food, it is an indication that our spirits are not free either. God indicates that there is a kind of fasting that leads to the freedom we really desire; the benefits are mental, emotional, spiritual and physical.

Follow the Divine Design!

What I've been saying, and will continue to say in this book, is that a loving Creator has left us an instruction book that wonderfully matches the design of His creation. As the apostle Paul wrote to the younger minister Timothy:

All scripture is given by inspiration of God, and is profitable. That the man of God may be perfect, throughly furnished unto all good works

(2 Tim. 3:16,17, KJV).

The primary message of both the Old and the New Testaments is salvation; and, as we have said, salvation comes through the blood sacrifice of the Messiah, not through eating habits.

Nevertheless, *a large portion of the Scripture focuses on commands, ordinances and statutes that show us how to live on this carefully designed earth.* Many of these passages pertain to subjects such as economics, law, government, interpersonal relationships, nutrition and health. The sacrifice of Jesus for our sins does not cancel the wisdom in these other teachings. As Paul said, they are still profitable (see 2 Tim. 3:16).

This book is not about miraculous intervention as an answer to prayer. Certainly God can do this in regard to illness when He chooses. This book is designed to help you discover the laws of God and apply them for health and wholeness. We will study both biblical and scientific laws that reveal how to recover and maintain health. You will see that the thoughts of our Creator are unparalleled in wisdom. You will experience firsthand what Florence Nightingale discovered: The laws of science are the thoughts of God.

2. Health with Obedience

Are we missing out on the health God promised His people by not following His laws?

Have you heard of the processionary caterpillar? It has an instinct that, although interesting, can be fatal. Processionary caterpillars have the habit of following their leader—whichever worm is walking in front of them. Their leader usually takes them to food—primarily the leaves of certain plants.

If you put these little critters on the rim of a cup, they will march one behind the other until a whole row of caterpillars form a circle. Once the leader starts out and the others begin to follow, the fateful stage is set. The entire herd will continue to walk round and round, until they die—even though many life-giving leaves can be found down in the cup itself.

Welcome to the Death March

People are sometimes similar to the processionary caterpillar. By uncritically following the lead of our culture, whether in the areas of truth, morals or health, we allow ourselves to be led to needless death.

My people are destroyed from lack of knowledge (Hos. 4:6)

The caterpillar in front of us is eating this or that, so we do the same, marching round and round the rim of the cup instead of dipping down and joyfully partaking of the food treasures God has created for us.

By modern definition, the disciplines and traditions of science limit themselves to discovering the laws of the material world, or what can be known from the five senses alone. According to this view—strictly speaking—science can say absolutely nothing either about the existence, or the nonexistence, of God. Neither can modern science say anything at all about morality, nor ethics, nor beauty, nor meaning in life. These self-imposed limits of modern science rule out discussion of the supernatural and anything else that cannot be measured.[1]

I take issue with this definition because it leaves much of reality out of the equation. A much more useful definition is provided by *Webster's Dictionary:*

> *Science is a systematized knowledge derived from observation, study and experimentation carried on in order to determine the nature of what is being studied.*

In this view of science, which is the classical view of science, the possibility of a Creator is not excluded from the start. In this view, if the evidence leads to a first cause for everything, then a possible Creator is an allowable subject for discussion. In this view, a scientist may do science, notice the wise and intricate hand of a Designer and ascribe glory to God, because all of creation tells forth the glory of God (see Ps. 19:1,2; Rom. 1:20). This definition has been almost totally excluded from academic institutions for several decades.[2] We have suffered greatly because of this redefinition of science, not just because of the spiritual effect of nonbelief, but because of the resulting widespread attitude that because there is no design to the universe, we human beings are the masters of our universe.

If there is no God, then there is no Designer to the universe; and if there is no Designer, there is no design. And if there is no design, then people and food as well came about as a result of random chance. In this scenario, there are absolutely no absolutes; people can do whatever they feel they have a right to do. Society has no basis or right on which to say heterosexual marriage is better than homosexual marriage, that raping the land is bad, no basis whatever for saying even that survival is an absolute good.

If there is no God, then we could not possibly thank the Creator for food. Food just "is." If food just "is," then in the name of progress scientists have every right to manipulate it, process it and alter it as suits the needs of the mass marketers.

Get in step, caterpillars. Left, left, left, right, left.

Dare to Be Different

People of faith are challenged:
> *"Do not follow the crowd in doing wrong"* (Exod. 23:2),
> and,
> *Do not imitate what is evil but what is good* (3 John 11).

Risk it, caterpillars. Get out of line. Read this book. Memorize The Three Principles:

- *Principle I:* Eat only substances God created for food.
- *Principle II:* As much as possible, eat foods as they were created—before they are changed or converted into something humans think might be better.
- *Principle III:* Avoid food addictions. Don't let any food or drink become your god.

You will be criticized. Other caterpillars want you to be just like them, but you will also be healthy.

Dare to Be Healthy

The aged apostle John wrote:
> *Dear friend, I pray that you may enjoy good health and that all may go well with you, even as your soul is getting along well* (3 John 2).

Would God have inspired John to

pray that we would enjoy good health—physically, mentally or spiritually—without giving us the required information?

The purpose of this book is to point you to the Creator's principles He provided to enable you to have good health; and to point out, if health problems do arise, biblical principles that can help you recover your health.

In doing so, I also want to encourage you to trust your soul personally to this God who loves you enough to provide instructions for taking care of your body.

The Bible is bold in promising us health according to His design. God's reputation is dependent on His promises to us for health:

> My son, attend to my words; incline thine ear unto my sayings. Let them not depart from thine eyes; keep them in the midst of thine heart. For they are life unto those that find them, and health to all their flesh (Prov. 4:20-22, KJV).

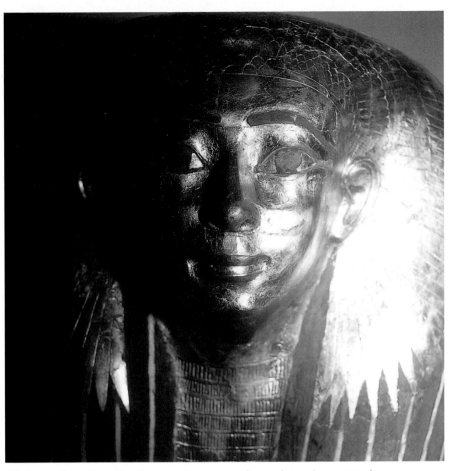

We know about Egyptian diseases from autopsies performed on mummies.

"None of These Diseases"

Several years ago, Dr. S. I. McMillen published a now-famous book by the title *None of These Diseases*.[3] He was right on target in calling our attention to the sound hygiene imbedded in the dietary laws of Scripture.

Along with Dr. McMillen, we have also noted the promise God made to the children of Israel: they would avoid the diseases that afflicted the Egyptians if they followed His directions (see Exod. 15:26).

What were the diseases God brought upon the Egyptians. Do they still exist today?

We have a clear idea of the Egyptian diseases from radiographs and autopsies performed on mummies by paleopathologist Marc A. Ruffer and others.[4] These studies show that many Egyptians had the same diseases that still cause illness today.

The most common affliction of the Egyptians appears to be vascular diseases that resulted in severely calcified arteries. Other common maladies included arthritis, tooth decay, infections, cancer, emphysema, tuberculosis, parasites, pneumonia and obesity. Childbirth deaths and infections after

birth were also fairly common.

Mummified Pharaohs often show the most advanced degenerative diseases. Historically, Pharaohs and other royalty (see 1 Kings 4:22ff.; Amos 6:4) were the only ones whose diets included large quantities of meat and other delicacies.

Modern research is showing that following the same ordinances God gave His people to protect them from the diseases of the Egyptians would help protect us from disease today. The list of modern causes of death is similar to the causes of death in those ancient days (see panel).

These modern diseases show the consequences of disobedience to God's ordinances.

Other Reasons We Die

Don't get sensitive. Not all disease is caused by disobedience.

Biblically, three kinds of illness are possible.

1. *Some sicknesses bring on death.*
   It is appointed unto men once to

Leading Causes of Death in the U.S. 1990[5]

1. Heart disease	**6.** Pneumonia
2. Cancer	**7.** Diabetes Mellitus
3. Cerebrovascular disease	**8.** Atherosclerosis
4. Chronic lung disease	**9.** Suicide
5. Accidents	**10.** HIV
	11. Hepatitis and cirrhosis

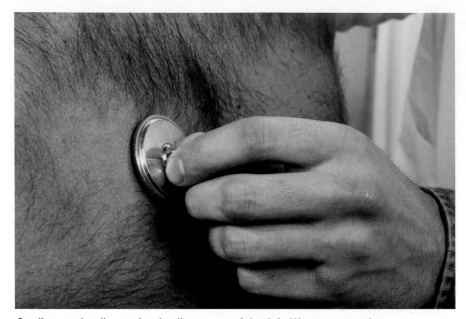

Cardiovascular disease is a leading cause of death in Western countries.

die, but after this the judgment (Heb. 9:27, KJV).

(We all get to have one such illness, like old age!)

2. *Some illnesses glorify God.* Strange, but true. Once Jesus and His disciples encountered a man who had been blind since birth. Like many people today, the disciples automatically associated all sickness with sin, so they asked Jesus:

Master, who did sin, this man, or his parents, that he was born blind? Jesus answered, Neither hath this man sinned, nor his parents: but that the works of God should be made manifest in him (John 9:2, KJV).

The apostle Paul's thorn in the flesh also served a similar purpose. When he asked unsuccessfully for God to remove it, God said:

My grace is sufficient for thee: for my strength is made perfect in weakness (2 Cor. 12:9, KJV).

3. *Some illness and death result from disobedience or ignorance.* As we have noted, God said:

My people are destroyed from lack of knowledge (Hos. 4:6).

And in Isaiah 1:19,20, God said, *If ye be willing and obedient, ye shall eat the good of the land: But if ye refuse and rebel, ye shall be devoured with the sword* (KJV).

The word for "devoured" here is from a Hebrew word that means drought, parching or decay caused by

cutting off by a sharp tool (i.e., amputation). The primary meaning here is that God will cut off Israel from Himself if they disobey; but it is also true that ignoring His commands regarding health can have a similar result physically. As an interesting parallel to this scriptural picture, most amputations today are caused by tissue deterioration caused by poor circulation. Strokes, heart attacks and hypertension have similar causes—most of which could be avoided by obeying His laws that are designed for our good health.

Prevention by Principle I

Let's apply Principle I to some specific illnesses to see what would happen if we ate only those foods God created for our health.

Hardening of the Arteries

Cardiovascular disease (arteriosclerosis, or hardening of the arteries—HA) is implicated in the first, third and eighth leading causes of death on the previous chart.

The first case of myocardial infarction was reported in the medical literature in 1906. Now the disease is so common that the smallest hospi-

tals have special units for such patients.

How does HA develop? To simplify a complex process, an "insult" or injury occurs in the intima (inner) layer of an artery. Toxins, viral infections, trauma, chemicals and radiation can cause injury to the inner layer of the artery. The artery responds by laying down cholesterol or a plaque to heal this insult. The plaque thickens the intima and narrows the lumen or opening of the artery. Turbulence begins and the flow of blood slows. Cells (platelets) clump together forming a clot, blocking the vessel.

If the coronary artery is blocked, a heart attack occurs. A blocked cerebral (brain) artery causes a stroke.

Hard animal fat has a fatty acid that is sticky and causes platelets to clump together. Most of the things we are warned to avoid in Scripture contribute to this disease.

Several years ago Dr. Ben Feingold withheld several foods, including fruits and vegetables, from the diets of hyperactive children because he believed the tiny amounts of aspirin in these foods caused their hyperactivity. Further research has exonerated or cleared these foods and aspirin as a cause of hyperactivity.[6]

We have learned that tiny amounts of aspirin inhibit the clumping of platelets. Taking an aspirin a day does decrease the incidence of heart attacks and even some strokes. Taking aspirin, however, increases the number of hemorrhagic strokes (bleeding into the brain).

Apparently produce such as fruits and vegetables has just the right amount of aspirin to prevent both kinds of strokes—unnecessary clotting and hemorrhagic strokes. Just three vegetables a day decrease the incidence of strokes and heart attacks by a significant amount.

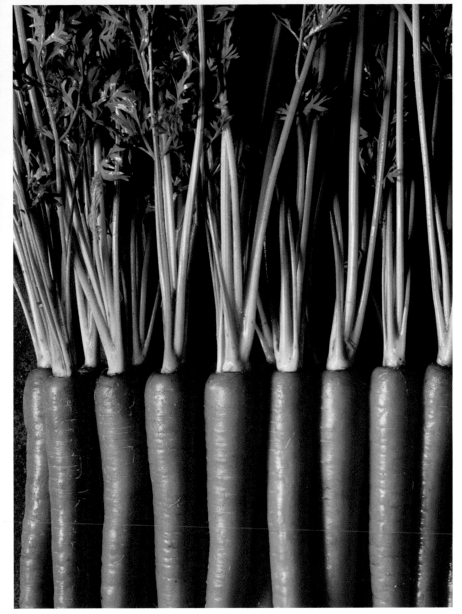

Fruits and vegetables have just the right amount of aspirin to prevent strokes.

We have also learned that vitamins C, E and B6, as well as linoleic acid—all essential nutrients—inhibit platelet clumping. It is interesting that onions, garlic, leeks, pineapples and mackerel (see chapter 3) do the same, and probably more efficiently.

Principle I and Cancer

In 1993, Dr. Michael Thun, and Dr. Peter Greenwald, Director of Cancer Prevention at the National Cancer Institute in Bethesda, Maryland, summarized separate studies on 635,000 Americans. Those Americans who consumed aspirin had a 40 percent lower incidence of colon, stomach and esophageal cancers. Dr. G. A. Burkhart confirmed these findings in a report about colon cancers in the *Annals of Internal Medicine* 1995.[7]

The safest way to intake aspirin at nontoxic levels is from the mainstays of God's created food. This one tiny ingredient in the things created for foods fights the first two causes of death in our country: vascular disease and cancer.

Recently, cancer has become the most common cause of death in the United States among people between the ages of 35 and 70. Deaths from cancer are increasing yearly and outstripping the aging rate of our population (*see panel on page 22*).

The University of Texas M. D. Anderson Hospital in Houston reported the relevant mechanics of the development of cancer. The following are the conclusions drawn:[9]

1. Certain "genotoxic events" such as radiation, chemicals or viruses actually change normal cells into abnormal or cancerous cells.

2. Certain "epigenetic events" either stimulate or impede the growth of abnormal cells.

All of the epigenetic factors that impede carcinogens and abnormal cell growth are found in the highest bioavailable forms in the substances God created for food (Principle I). (Bioavailable refers to the rate at which an element enters the blood stream and is utilized by specific organs or tissues.)

Also, many genotoxic substances (viruses and chemicals) are transmitted by eating toxic flesh such as scavengers, the blood of any animal or the fat of cattle, sheep or goat—items God did not intend for us to eat.

Other infectious agents that lead to cancer are also rapidly passed along from person to person by breaking God's law on monogamous sex (see chapter 4).

Principle I and Diabetes

There are two types of diabetes. Type one is juvenile onset diabetes, which is insulin dependent. Type two is adult onset diabetes, which may be controlled by oral medications, weight loss, insulin or diet.

Type one diabetes usually appears in children. The causes of juvenile diabetes are difficult to ascertain. It frequently occurs in families, which has caused many people to conclude that diabetes is inherited. Opposing evidence shows that juvenile diabetes is more likely caused by a slow virus.

The mechanism for developing juvenile diabetes occurs when the virus somehow confuses the immune system into destroying islet cells of the pancreas. The islet cells produce insulin, which controls blood sugar.

Viruses may cause many other chronic illnesses as well. Included in this list are multiple sclerosis, Lou Gehrig's Disease (amyotropic lateral sclerosis), shingles, some cancers, hardening of the arteries, systemic lupus, rheumatoid arthritis, Alzheimer's disease and many others.

In many cases, these viruses are

passed through foods and activities that are forbidden by the divine design. Viral hepatitis, which leads to cirrhosis, liver failure and liver cancer, is transmitted through eating shellfish and blood. Promiscuous sex and other biblical forms of uncleanness also result in viral transmission of hepatitis as well as other viral diseases.

Do these lifestyles tend to be learned in families? Yes.

Do families become exposed to the same virus? Yes.

One contaminated piece of unclean flesh could expose everyone. A few members of the family may get sick, although because it is a slow virus, the onset of the disease may not occur for weeks or years. Many will say the disease is inherited; but it may well be a case of bad habits rather than bad genes.

Some diseases are inherited, but blaming parents for bad choices is a cop-out. We all inherit one trait that is devastating: our desire to do things our own way (our sin nature).

The divine design, which requires grace (power and desire given by God to follow the divine design) and discipline, will protect us from many sorrows.

Studies have indicated that insulin requirements in diabetics will drop as a person begins eating high-fiber foods such as beans, oats, grains, vegetables and fruits.

E. Cheraskin and William Ringsdorf at the University of Alabama and Dr. James Anderson at the University of Kentucky have been able to help relieve juvenile diabetics from taking insulin by putting them on diets of pure water, fresh vegetables and fruit. This diet is not only what the doctor ordered, but based on foods the Creator designed.[10]

Other diabetics have even been able to stop using insulin completely by following this kind of diet.[11] I believe many cases of juvenile diabetes could be aborted if this kind of diet were followed soon after the onset of the disease. This would be an interesting research project.

In addition to insulin deficiency in diabetics, the enzymes produced by the pancreas are also deficient. These enzymes are designed to digest the foods. Without these enzymes, foods may not be well digested. So diabetics

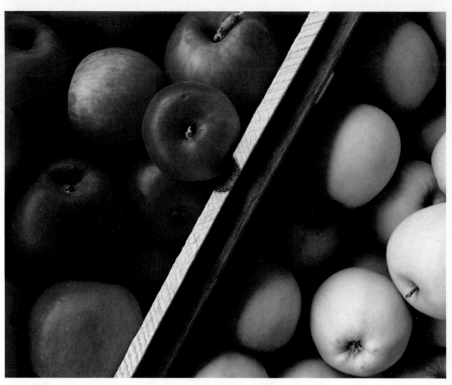

The diabetic can be helped by eating what God has provided for food.

need foods loaded with nutrients, as well as some dietary supplements.

These nutrients are best found in fresh vegetables such as sprouts, whole-grain bread, fruits and other foods that have high fiber content. The diabetic can be helped by eating what God has provided for food. These foods will need to be eaten before being changed into nutrient deficient products.

Another helpful activity for diabetics is exercise. Exercise lowers the insulin requirements.

Exploring Principle II

Principle II and Cancer

Overwhelming scientific evidence shows the wisdom of eating foods as God created them—before they are changed or converted into something humans thinks might be better.

Dr. Michail J. Wargovich of M. D. Anderson Hospital in Houston states that scientists are looking at several isolated chemicals that seek to stop cancer from developing even where a carcinogen is present. He reports:

In the last three to four years we've found that fruits *and* vegetables [author's emphasis] *contain a variety of powerful chemicals which interact and bind to chemical carcinogens, rendering them inactive. Some of these chemicals might also interfere with the metabolism of carcinogens rendering them inactive. Some of these chemicals might also interfere with the metabolism of carcinogens in the liver.*[12]

The foods God created for us not only minister health to us, but they also actually heal! That should be no surprise in view of Exodus 15:26 (KJV):

I am the Lord that healeth thee.
"Heal" here is from the Hebrew word *raphah*, which means to *mend, cure* or *repair.*

Principle II Warnings

The three major chemical groups Dr. Wargovich is studying are sulfides, indoles and phenols. Sulfides are found in garlic and onion, and indoles are found in vegetables such as broccoli, cauliflower, brussels sprouts and cabbage. Phenols can be found in almost all raw fruits and vegetables.

According to Wargovich, the key word is "raw." Cooking destroys these anticarcinogens. Dr. Wargovich points out that the background for his research lies in studies of Western diet trends. Cancer rates differ among dif-

1. *Red dye No. 2.* The good news is that this substance, which has been linked to cancer in test animals, has now been removed from the market in the United States, and has been replaced with red dye No. 40. The bad news is that red dye No. 40 is also a suspected carcinogen.

2. *DES.* This is a synthetic hormone used in chicken and cattle feed. It has been linked to carcinoma of the cervix.

3. *Sodium nitrite.* This substance, found in cured meats such as hot dogs, sausage and bologna, forms nitrosamines, which are potent carcinogens.

4. *Tobacco products.*

5. *Smog.*

6. *Cyclamates and saccharin.*

7. *Hexachlorophene,* widely used in cosmetics, deodorants and other toilet articles, and as soap in hospitals.

8. *Strontium No. 90 and iodine No. 131.* These radioactive fallouts from atomic tests are found in our food chain, particularly in cows' milk.

9. *Cadmium.* This substance— from sources such as automobile exhaust, fertilizers and industrial waste—pollutes soil and water, and is found heavily concentrated at dangerous levels in shellfish.

10. *Drugs and environmental chemicals.* We are now exposed to some 7,600 chemicals in our foods. Many that have been tested are thought to be carcinogens; and most of the chemicals to which we are exposed have never been tested. These chemicals are found in our food, cosmetics, insecticides, pest repellents and defoliants.

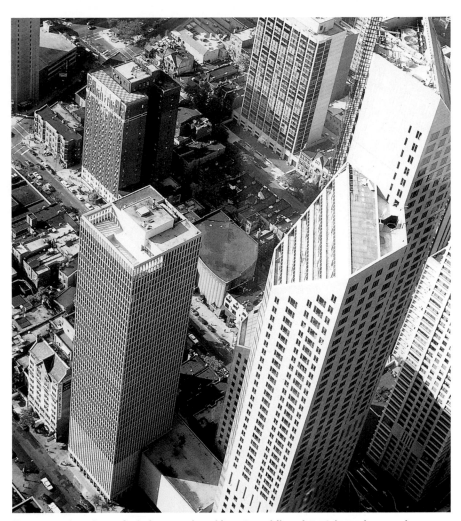

Downtown heat haze. Cadmium, produced in automobile exhaust, is a prime carcinogen.

ferent societies, and 70 to 80 percent of the cancers are probably caused by factors in food.

His research implies that human processing, preserving and polluting habits remove most of the protective and healing factors from what God created for food.

The panel lists some examples of epigenetic or genotoxic factors that should raise a warning flag:

It should be noted that chemicals are absorbed through the skin as well as through our digestive tracts. As you may know, many drugs are now administered by skin patches.

In summary, the factors that prevent and fight cancer cells are found in the things created for food that have not been processed or contaminated with any additional chemicals. From 80 to 90 percent of our nuts, vegetables and fruits should be eaten raw, and in their unprocessed forms. Sprouted grains and beans are excellent. Legumes and breads eaten soon after cooking are great. Avoid rancid breads and oils. Olive oil and 3-omega oils are great.

Principle II and Adult Onset Diabetes

Adult onset diabetes seems to be caused by eating refined and toxic foods and by a low physical activity level. One good example of this can be seen on the island of Nauru in the Pacific Ocean, where the economy once afforded the natives few luxuries. They raised most of their own foods on the island, and had few delicacies. They were generally healthy people and only one small hospital served the entire population.

Their lives changed when phosphorus was found in great quantities on the island. That discovery transformed the island's inhabitants into extremely wealthy people. They began to import much of the world's refined delicacies. Within 30 years after this lifestyle change, a 30 percent occurrence of adult onset diabetes developed. No measurable diabetes had been known previously. Now, after 40 years, 65 percent of the adult population has diabetes.[13]

Dr. James Anderson at the University of Kentucky, attributes this epidemic of diabetes on Nauru and other places throughout the world to lifestyle changes. No evidence suggests that the disease in these instances stems from a viral infection such as that seen in juvenile kind of diabetes.

Although genetic as well as environmental factors may also be involved, genetic weaknesses never manifest themselves until processed foods and delicacies are involved.[14] Those Nauruans who still live on farms and grow their own food remain free of the diabetes epidemic.

These Nauruan people illustrate Principle II very well. Although diabetes is their most common disease now, researchers predict that heart attacks, strokes, cancer and hypertension will soon be prevalent among these people, who were formerly healthy, but now are wealthy. Fortunately (really) they can afford the best medical facilities in the Pacific.

The American Diabetic Association, after much research by Dr. James Anderson, finally recommends such "Principle II" approaches as avoiding overly processed white flour, and eating plenty of fresh vegetables, fruits and other high-fiber foods such as legumes and whole-grain breads.[15] Yet it is amazing how many adult onset diabetics refuse to avoid white flour, much less the other recommendations. They seem to be saying, "I'd rather do it my way." They seem to be waiting for some miracle or some pill to heal them.

Hundreds of case histories support the reversal of adult onset diabetes by proper diet. Millions would recover if they would eat according to the three principles in Scripture previously discussed.

A six-year-old boy had intermittent high blood sugars of 360 mg/cc, and +4 (high) urine sugars during a 30-day period. Several months of a strict rotation diet of fresh vegetables,

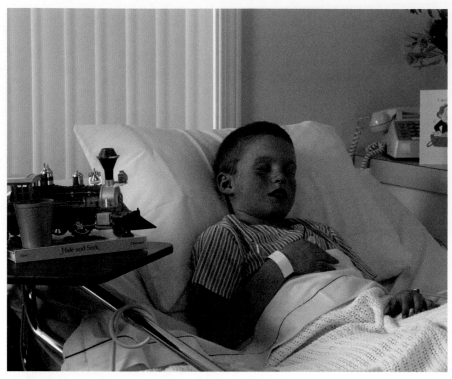

A six-year-old diabetic was treated with a strict diet of fruit, vegetables and grains.

fruits, whole-grain breads, legumes and some meats resulted in normal blood sugars for the following 18 years. The diet was not given for the purpose of treating the apparent diabetes. The diabetes was an incidental finding. Apparently the nutrients in these things created for food were enough to prevent the progressive destruction of the pancreas.

If the body's immune system is attacking its own pancreatic cells, could healthful nutrients allow it to correct itself? I believe they can!

A modern approach to reversing insulin-dependent diabetes is to stun the immune system so that it will not destroy the pancreas. It has worked in some cases, but, in a weakened immune system, the patients become susceptible to many other diseases.

If you are a diabetic, listen to your physicians. They will offer many ways to help you control your blood sugars to help you feel better. They will suggest medications to help you avoid crises and prevent some of the complications of diabetes, such as kidney failure. If you will follow the diet discussed here, physicians will also enjoy you as a patient, and be encouraged by your wanting to do what is best for your health. Some will also marvel at how long you can go on without

crisis or complications. Your visits will be more infrequent.

Eat real chemical-free, unprocessed food. Exercise, and drink clean chemical-free beverages (such as pure water), and your physicians will think they are geniuses and will brag about how well you are doing.

Exploring Principle III

Principle III, please remember, is that we should not allow ourselves to elevate any food or other substance to the level of a god, as in the case of food addictions. Each of the most common substances to which people become addicted yields not health, but health hazards.

Alcohol yields cancers of the liver, esophagus, mouth and pancreas.[16]

Cigarettes yield lung and bladder cancers.

Fats (hard animal fats and hydrogenated liquid fats) yield colon and breast cancers.

Salt in bacon, ham and sausage can initiate esophagus and stomach cancers (although I suspect these toxic meats are more risky than the salt: see chapter 8.)

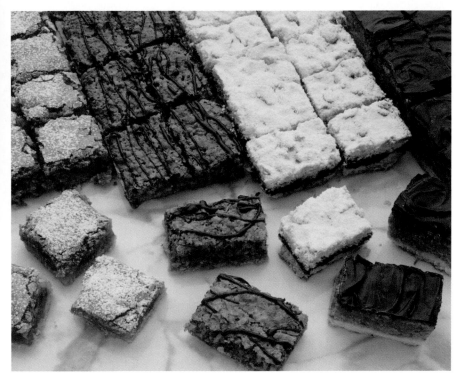

Most of the foods to which people become addicted are delicacies.

Twenty years ago, an expert committee convened by the World Health Organization (WHO) recognized that most cancers were related to lifestyle and environmental factors, and that the majority of human cancer is therefore potentially preventable. The committee cited causes of cancer, including natural carcinogens, viruses, nutritional factors, reproductive activity and other personal behavioral factors.

Such "Personal behavioral factors" involve morals, forgiveness, the golden rule and so on. Does the Bible speak to such politically incorrect ideas? Smile and read on. It will be good for you!

Intermittent fasts supplemented with organic, freshly squeezed juices from green or yellow vegetables and fruits help ensure that we will not become addicted either to the common substances previously listed or to any other food substance.

For the Bible's warnings against the highly addictive substance of alcohol, see chapter 12.

Lifestyle warnings could certainly include addicting and mind-altering drugs such as cocaine and marijuana.[17] The chemicals in marijuana that cause problems in judgment will give a desired "high" for only a few hours. Tests reveal, however, that this drug may still cause problems in discrimination and judgment for up to three months after a single joint has been smoked.

Food addictions or maladaptive reactions are described in the book *Brain Allergies* by William Philpott, M.D. His evidence would indicate that Principle III (fasting and avoiding addictions) probably would reduce the incidence of accidents, psychological disorders and physical illnesses.[18] Substances such as caffeine, sugar, salt, fat, dyes and MSG (monosodium glutamate) all have the potential to alter our judgment and certainly make us irritable.

A ranch in South Texas has taken in young incorrigibles for years. They begin feeding the delinquents only the foods God has created for our use. The ranch raises most of what is eaten. The camp allows no cigarettes, sugar, cokes, candy and so on. Within a short time the youth become reasonable, disciplined workers.[19]

Although avoiding addictive substances is only one factor in this camp's success with these troubled youngsters, the authorities consider eating real food vitally important. Many others have documented similar cases with incorrigibles.[20]

Warnings from Scripture

Most of the foods to which people become addicted are delicacies—rare and in some cases costly substances that in earlier times were reserved for royalty. Look at the following passages from Proverbs 23, which relate to health and also warn against being negatively swayed by those of influence.

When you sit to dine with a ruler, note well what is before you (v. 1).
Put a knife to your throat if you are given to gluttony (v. 2).
Do not crave his delicacies, for that food is deceptive (v. 3).
Do not eat the food of a stingy man, do not crave his delicacies (v. 6).

We can't help but note the implication of addiction in the word "crave."

Psalm 141:4 links food delicacies that can produce craving with evil behavior—just as in today's world:

Let not my heart be drawn to what is evil, to take part in wicked deeds with men who are evildoers; let me not eat of their delicacies.

These warnings do not appear to be subtle. The delicacies of the rulers described in these Scriptures were the ancient equivalent of sugars and white flour; things only royalty could afford in those days.

The Point of It All

Diabetes, cancer and heart disease can be prevented by obeying the Divine Design, and they can be caused by ignoring that design.

The treatments utilizing the Divine Design can delay the complications of these diseases, and often cure them as well.[21]

The Three Principles are found to be true:

1. Eat the things God created for food, and avoid everything else.
2. Eat the things created for food before they are changed into nutrient deficient or toxic products.
3. Avoid addictions. Intermittent fasting will help.

We are not saying that it is always easy to attain health with obedience. In 1 Corinthians 9:27 the apostle Paul said:

I buffet my body and make it my slave (NASB).

Let's face it: the word "buffet" in this passage isn't pronounced buff-FAY, and Paul isn't telling us to eat a tableful of delicacies. Sorry—he's advising us to discipline our bodies!

Blessings

God promises us countless blessings that more than offset the difficulties and discipline of obedience.

Bless the Lord, O my soul, and forget not all his benefits: who forgiveth all thine iniquities; who healeth all thy diseases; who redeemeth thy life from destruction; who crowneth thee with lovingkindness and tender mercies; who satisfieth thy mouth with good things; [such as foods—RR] *so that thy youth is renewed like the eagle's* (Ps. 103:2-5, KJV).

"I am the Lord your God, who teaches you what is best for you, who directs you in the way you should go. If only you had paid attention to my commands, your peace would have been like a river, your righteousness like the waves of the sea" (Isa. 48:17,18).

Modern examples of recovery from various diseases are numerous when these principles are followed. What about hypertension, arthritis, scleroderma, lupus and so on? Sure. It can be done.[22]

As mentioned earlier, physicians who study the aged tell us that we should live for 120 years when we follow a proper diet and exercise. Why do we live only 70 to 75 years, and the last 14 or so years we are usually in poor health? Does disobedience shorten our days? (*see* Ps. 90:7-10).

And Curses

Conversely, the Bible is clear about the consequences of disobedience:

If you do not carefully follow all the words of this law, which are written in this book, and do not revere this glorious and awesome name—the Lord your God—the Lord will send fearful plagues on you and your descendants, harsh and prolonged disasters, and severe and lingering illnesses. He will bring upon you all the diseases of Egypt that you dreaded, and they will cling to you (Deut. 28:58-60).

The words "cling" and "linger" are terms that accurately describe the chronic illnesses many of us have accepted without much resistance, and do not attempt to obey God's laws for good health.

How much happier and healthier we would be if we paid attention to God's design!

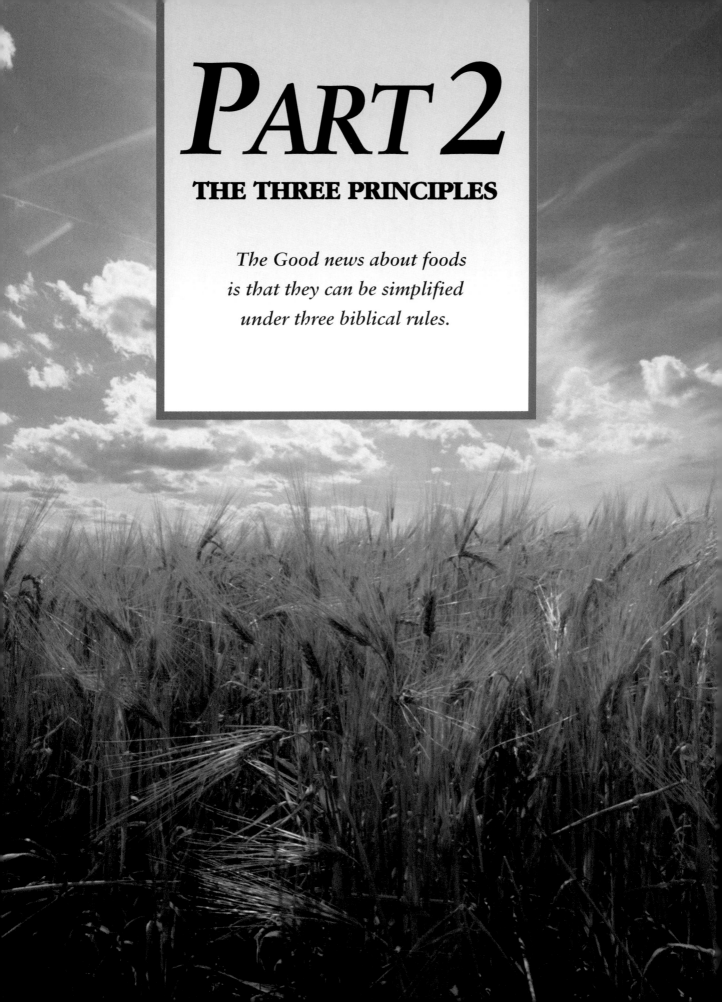

PART 2

THE THREE PRINCIPLES

*The Good news about foods
is that they can be simplified
under three biblical rules.*

3. Principle I

Eat the Foods God Created for You

Question: What's the best medicine for continued good health?
Answer: Food!

Have you ever played the game called Treasure Hunt? A list of things to find is given the players, along with a few clues, and the search begins. There are many varieties of the game, and all of them are fun and challenging.

For me, however, the best treasure hunt is finding healthful food at each meal. When I find it, my rule is to eat it with joy and vigor. This chapter will give you many clues for applying Principle I of The Three Principles—discovering what God has created specifically for food. Start your treasure hunt. Cheer yourself or your family on when you find a treasure to enjoy. It will be great for you!

What Is God's Design for Food?

"Food for the stomach and the stomach for food"—but God will destroy them both (1 Cor. 6:13).

What you consume as food is probably based on what your family enjoys, what advertisers promote or what fad is "in" at a given time. What the government promotes, and social and economic factors, are also influential. An example of the latter is serving meat with each meal, which became a sign of being a good provider during the depression of the late '20s and '30s—a

tradition that has continued for many until this day.

The word translated "food" in the New International Version of the Bible, or "meat" in the King James Version (KJV), comes from the Greek word *bromah*. In the Old Testament, *lechem*, the Hebrew word for food, is often translated "meat" in the KJV and "food" in most modern translations.

The Good News About Food

Spiritually, the gospel is "salvation." (Look in appendix 3 for what the Creator has done for you to have a personal relationship with Him.)

Mentally, the gospel promotes a sound mind. (Forgiveness, love, service and healthful eating are great for our minds.)

Physically, the good news is that God has provided many great things for food.

Allow me to suggest three boundaries in Scripture within which we can identify what God intended for us to eat.

1. When the Designer calls an item food.

Then God said, "I give you every seed-bearing plant on the face of the whole earth and every tree that has fruit with seed in it. They will be for your food" (Gen. 1:29).
And you will eat the plants of the field (3:18).

Pulses and nuts for sale at the traditional market at Beersheba, Israel.

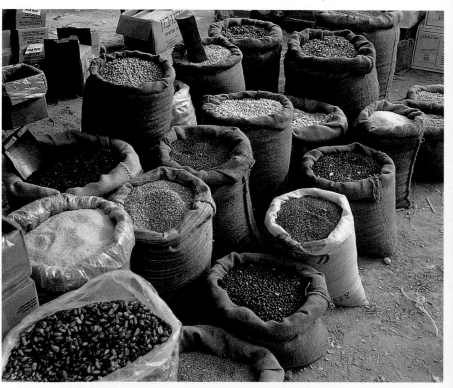

2. When God brings items to His people as a gift.

Also the food I provided for you— the fine flour, olive oil and honey I gave you to eat— declares the Sovereign Lord (Ezek. 16:19).

3. If Jesus ate or served an item.

Then he took the seven loaves and the fish, and when he had given thanks, he broke them and gave them to the disciples, and they in turn to the people (Matt. 15:36).

The box on page 32 gives a list of foods that Scripture guarantees are designed for health and that may be enjoyed. They were created for food. (Keep in mind Principle II, however: If these foods are altered, they may lose many of their benefits.)

These foods are gold mines filled with essentials for healthy cells. They probably have millions of healthful components we have not yet identified or don't know how they function. Please enjoy them. They are better than medicine. (This list isn't exhaustive, as the following information will reveal.)

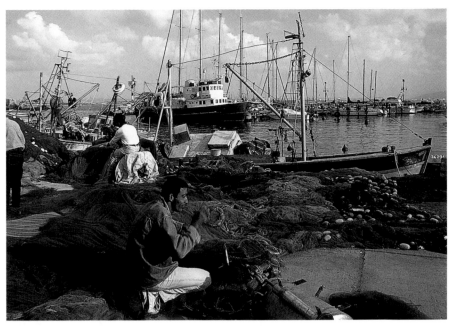

Israeli fishermen mend their nets before setting sail for another harvest of the sea.

Believe It or Not

On an island off the southern tip of Korea live a group of women who eat a potion made primarily of pulverized locusts, grasshoppers and honey. They live as long or longer than any people on earth, and have little or no disease.

Maybe John the Baptist was a health nut:

And the same John had his raiment of camel's hair, and a leathern girdle about his loins; and his meat was locusts and wild honey (Matt. 3:4, KJV).

Don't lose your head about eating locusts.

Gene DeFoliart, editor of *The Food Insects Newsletter*, says, "They're better than what you're going to get at your average fast-food restaurant."[1]

Warnings Against Some Foods

In the Old Testament, God commanded the Israelites not to eat some items.

Even today, though not on a spiritual level, these commands are still relevant for our health. These foods will be covered more extensively in later chapters.

"Do not eat any of the fat of cattle, sheep, or goats" (Lev. 7:23).
You must not eat the blood; pour it out on the ground like water (Deut. 12:16).
"Do not eat the meat of an animal torn by wild beasts." Do not eat road kill [author's modern-day translation] (Exod. 22:31).
"You must distinguish between the unclean and the clean, between living creatures that may be eaten and those that may not be eaten" (Lev. 11:47).

Puffer fish or file fish have poisonous flesh that will make you sick or kill you if eaten.[2]

Remember, I am not calling for a return to the old law for spiritual benefit; but I am asking that we recognize the health benefits in these ancient commands. God cared for His Old Testament people through them, and He will take care of us if we observe them, too.

Expanding the Lists

Neither the healthful nor the unhealthful foods on the list are all inclusive. Many plants fit into the categories of Genesis 1:29a: wheat, rice, oats, barley, millet, rye and other grains; legumes of all kinds (e.g., peas, beans); bush and vine-bearing fruits and vegetables (melons, grapes, berries, squash, tomatoes, eggplant, cucumbers, etc.).

In Genesis 1:29b (KJV), God also gave us:

every tree, in the which is the fruit of a tree yielding seed; to you it shall be for meat [food].

This includes every conceivable fruit (apples, pears, apricots, plums, mangoes, avocado, etc.), as well as all nuts, both large and small (coconuts, walnuts, almonds, cashews, etc.).

The Adequacy of Approved Food

Now let's analyze God's generous provision to see if it contains adequate amounts of the three main food types: *carbohydrates*, *proteins* and *fats*.

Fiber-rich carbohydrates are present in abundance in all plant foods.

How about protein? All plants have some protein, but legumes, nuts and grains have the highest proportions. By mixing the various plant foods, all the essential amino acids are present, making "complete" proteins.

Guaranteed for Health

The following is a list of foods that Scripture guarantees are designed for health and that may be enjoyed. They were created for food. (Keep in mind Principle II, however: If these foods are altered, they may lose many of their benefits.)

These foods are gold mines filled with essentials for healthy cells. They probably have millions of healthful components we have not yet identified or don't know how they function. Please enjoy them. They are better than medicine. (This list isn't exhaustive.)

almonds	Genesis 43:11
barley	Judges 7:13
beans	Ezekiel 4:9
beef	1 Kings 4:22,23
bread	1 Samuel 17:17
broth	Judges 6:19
cakes	2 Samuel 13:8 (KJV)
cheese	Job 10:10
cucumbers, onions, leeks, melons, garlic	Numbers 11:5
curds of cow's milk	Deuteronomy 32:14
figs	Numbers 13:23
fish	Matthew 7:10
fowl	1 Kings 4:23
fruit	2 Samuel 16:2
game	Genesis 25:28
goat's milk	Proverbs 27:27
grain	Ruth 2:14
veal	Genesis 18:7,8
vegetables	Proverbs 15:17
grapes	Deuteronomy 23:24
grasshoppers, locusts, crickets	Leviticus 11:22 (The finicky have something to fuss about.)
herbs	Exodus 12:8
honey	Isaiah 7:15
lentils	Genesis 25:34
meal	Matthew 13:33 (KJV)
nuts	Genesis 43:11
oil	Proverbs 21:17
olives	Deuteronomy 28:40
pomegranates	Numbers 13:23
quail	Numbers 11:32
raisins	2 Samuel 16:1
salt	Job 6:6
sheep	Deuteronomy 14:4
sheep's milk	Deuteronomy 32:14
spices	Genesis 43:11
vinegar	Numbers 6:3
wild honey	Psalm 19:10

What about fats? Nuts are the richest fat-containing plants; the fats in plants are healthful when eaten in moderation; and no plant food contains cholesterol.

Dr. Ethyl Nelson proposes many interesting theories about which foods are best suited for us.[3] Not only is she a board-certified pathologist, but she also gained much of her insight from her 25 years of service as a missionary, which enabled her to compare the Western world's diet to the diet of Adam and Eve in the garden.

In Genesis 3, note that after Adam and Eve fell into sin God ordered a dietary addition: "You shall eat the herb of the field" (v. 18, NKJV). This was the food previously designated for the animals. These were herbs without seed in them, such as lettuce, cabbage, broccoli, cauliflower, spinach, asparagus, etc., and the tubers (yams, potatoes, carrots, beets, etc.).[4] After the devastating flood wiped out all vegetation, God gave another decree regarding diet:

"Every moving thing that lives shall be food for you. I have given you all things, even as the green herbs. But you shall not eat flesh with its life, that is, its blood" (9:3,4, NKJV).

Apparently, in the beginning people were to be complete vegetarians. Was this an adequate diet? Obviously yes, for most of these antediluvians reportedly had life spans approaching 1,000 years.

Even after the flood man was not to eat every kind of meat. What about selecting the animals that entered the ark?

"You shall take with you seven each of every clean animal, a male and his female; two each of animals that are unclean, a male and his female; also seven each of the birds of the air, male and female, to keep the species alive on the face of all the earth" (7:2,3, NKJV).

After the flood:

Noah built an altar to the Lord, and took of every clean animal and of every clean bird, and offered burnt offerings on the altar (8:20, NKJV).

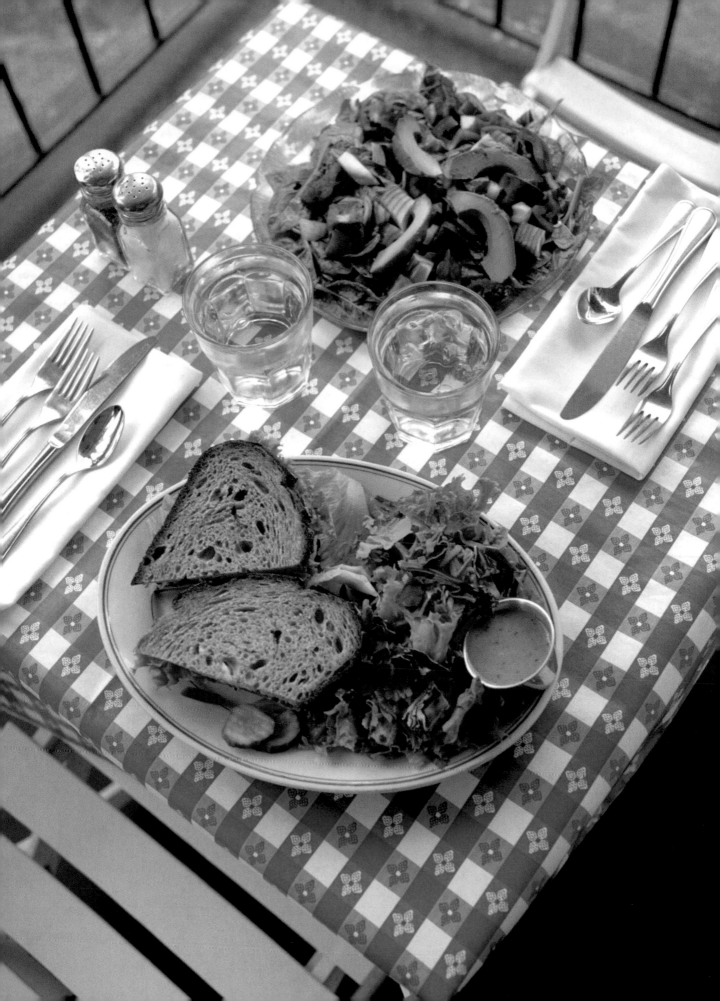

One each of the seven clean animals and birds was used for an offering, leaving three pairs of every kind. As Dr. Nelson argues, if any unclean animal had been eaten (of which there was but one pair) the species would have become extinct.[5] Therefore, Noah's family must have eaten only the clean animals (see the designations in Leviticus 11).

The other restriction was that no blood was to be eaten (Gen. 9:4). Blood is the body's transport system, carrying in it all waste products for disposal.

Adam may have received this message at the time of the Fall. No one really knows when humans started eating flesh, but Adam's rebellious nature suggests that he ate what he wanted (i.e., the fruit of the tree of knowledge of good and evil).

The best justification for eating meat is probably that Jesus ate fish and lamb, foods approved in Leviticus and Deuteronomy. Preparation and contamination of meat, however, present real problems for the meat eater today. (Remember Principle II about eating foods before humans have "fixed" them; see also chapter 8.)

God Knew What People Needed

To maintain good health, certain things must be present and in proper balance (*see panel in next column*).

These items must come from outside the body. Many recent studies prove that the bioavailability of these essentials are found in their maximum concentrations in the food approved by God for the Israelites.

It is generally agreed that degenerative diseases can result from deficiencies of any of these factors. If these deficiencies are not corrected, illness or death will result.

Excesses and imbalance of any of these nutrients may also cause disease. It is estimated that 60 percent of the population ingest too much of one fatty acid—(linoleic)—and 95 percent ingest too little of the other essential fatty acid—(linolenic) (*see column 3*).

Many believe that simply adding additional fiber to our diets prevents

Essentials for healthy living

1. The essential amino acids from proteins
2. Vitamins
3. Minerals
4. Two essential fatty acids
5. Unrefined carbohydrates
6. Unknown food factors
7. Water
8. Oxygen
9. Light ("God saw that the light was good" [Gen. 1:4]. "When Jesus spoke again to the people, he said, 'I am the light of the world. Whoever follows me will never walk in darkness, but will have the light of life.'" [John 8:12].)

most of these diseases (see the following information).[7]

If our cells are receiving the essentials for health, these diseases will not occur. Remember the Hunza people (chapter 1)?

Unknown Food Factors

Thousands of unknown factors exist in food. You may remember when fiber gained the spotlight a few years ago. Dr. Denis Burkitt, a missionary surgeon in Africa, brought fiber to the world's attention at a time when fiber was being removed from the diet of patients who suffered from ulcers, hemorrhoids and colitis.

Dr. Burkitt noticed that he rarely had to operate on natives who ate the traditional high-fiber diet. On the other hand, the British population in his area who ate refined food were frequently brought to surgery, and were afflicted with all of the top 10 diseases.

The Africans who attended school in England soon were needing surgery

Other than these essentials, what else is available from the foods approved by God for the Israelites? First, let's look at the top 10 leading causes of hospitalizations or insurance claims for the United States in 1990.

1. **Obesity.** This was not even a medical term 200 years ago. It is a modern disease. Eating less, and eating plenty of fiber, whole grains, vegetables and legumes without animal fat and heavily processed oils can prevent or cure obesity.

2. **Diabetes.** No cases were found in the Nauru Islands in 1955. Now, 40 years after changing to refined foods, 65 percent of the population is diabetic.

3. **Hemorrhoids, varicose veins.**[6]

4. **Heart attacks,** which were a medical oddity in the 1920s. It is still rare in Japan.

5. **Diverticulosis** and **diverticulitis** (*colitis*).

6. **Cancer.**

7. **Peptic ulcer.**

8. **Hiatal hernia.**

9. **Appendicitis.**

10. **Gallstones.**[7]

for appendicitis, hemorrhoids, ulcers and gallstones. They were enjoying processed foods without fiber.

Are other previously unknown food factors still being discovered? Yes! Where are they found? They are found in the foods approved by God. Many of the new factors are called phytochemicals and antioxidants:

1. Sulforaphane hinders the initiation phase of cancer. It is found in most vegetables such as broccoli, kale and onions.

2. Beta-carotene. An antioxidant

that destroys "free radicals" that attack all cells, leading to destructive processes. These are found in highest concentrations in yellow and green vegetables or fruits. They protect against lung cancer and many other of the diseases previously listed in our top 10 list.

3. Indole-3-Carbinol. Dr. Jon Michnovicz of the Institute of Hormone Research in New York City states that this phytochemical found in grains breaks down hormones that stimulate breast cancer growth.

4. Polyphenols, found in green teas.

5. Limonene in citrus fruits.

6. Quercetin in grapes, found in high concentrations in grape juice and lesser amounts in red wines. Polyphenols, limonene and quercetin all protect us against hardening of the arteries, which can lead to strokes, heart attacks and other diseases.

Food for Created Beings

Why do foods approved by God in the Old Testament suit us so well? And why do humans enjoy them so much? Let me describe a single aspect of the Creation issue that I believe points to a Creator as the answer to both questions.

Living proteins contain 22 amino acids. Scientists have learned that the body itself produces only 14 of them. The remaining eight that are equally essential for healthful living must therefore be eaten. Amino acids are the building blocks for proteins, which include hormones, structural proteins and enzymes. These specific entities are necessary for life.

Each enzyme promotes a particular chemical process in the living cell. The human body contains millions of precisely designed enzymes. The sequence of the 22 amino acids and the length of the amino acids chain determine the function of a particular protein.

Living proteins vary in length from 23 specifically sequenced amino acids in the hormone ACTH to several hundred thousand amino acids in hemoglobin. The probability that amino acids would get together in the right sequence purely by chance is

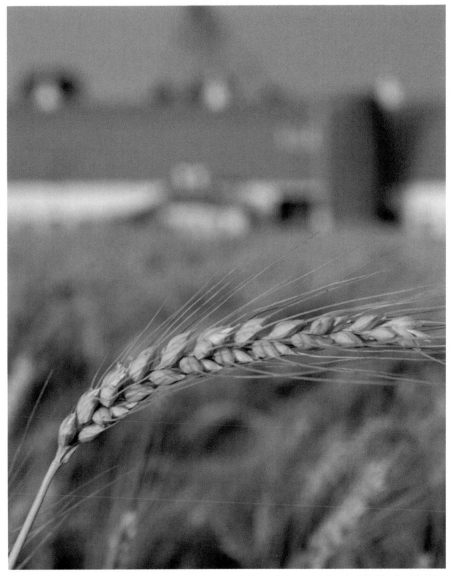

'The food I provided for you—the fine flour. . .' says the sovereign Lord' (Ezek. 16:19).

nonexistent. The nucleus of each cell contains very complex DNA molecules, which are coded with information to place amino acids in the proper order.

Living proteins are formed by DNA in the cells. For DNA to reproduce or function, a full complement of proteins is necessary. That means the very first cells required fully developed systems of proteins and DNA. The design had to be complete in the beginning. Time, regardless of how long, would be detrimental to chance development because proteins are destroyed by exposure to heat or oxygen. The proteins would be destroyed before they would be functional.

Dr. Carl Sagan, a leading teacher of

random evolution, estimates that the chance of life evolving on earth is 1 followed by 2 billion zeros. Great faith is needed to believe in Dr. Sagan's inconceivable theory. Dr. Emil Borel (an expert in mathematical probability) formulated this irrefutable law more than a century ago:

The occurrence of any event where the chances are beyond one followed by 50 zeros is an event which we can state with certainty will never happen, no matter how much time is allotted and no matter how many conceivable opportunities could exist for the event to take place.[8]

These observations about the formation of a cell point to a careful

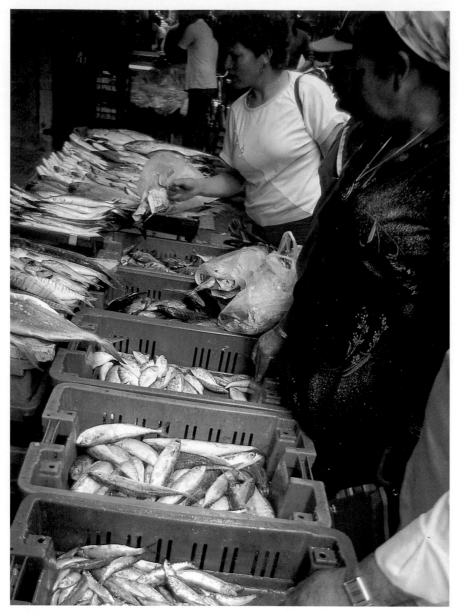

Locally caught fish for sale in the busy food market in Bethlehem, Israel.

design. Where there is a design there must be a designer. Does this Designer give us instructions about how to keep those cells healthy? Yes. And who can advise us better?

Do governments, the Food and Drug Administration, the American Medical Association, *The Ladies Home Journal,* the Mayo Clinic, Dr. Ruth or even Mom have more wisdom than the Designer, who built these complex structures for life?

Relax. Wise people will follow the Divine Design for health. If we were all wise, we would rarely need doctors—and the government could afford health care benefits for everyone! We would all put ourselves under the care of Him who brought Israel out of Egypt, having "not one feeble person among their tribes" (Ps. 105:37, KJV).

I wonder if the diet in Egypt had anything to do with it.

We [Israelites] remember the fish, which we did eat in Egypt freely; the cucumbers, and the melons, and the leeks, and the onions, and the garlick (Num. 11:5, KJV)

Doctors can relax. Given our fallen world, not enough people will ever be wise enough to follow the Divine Design and cause health care professionals to be put out of business.

4. Principle II

Don't Alter God's Design

"He loves me, he loves me not. Loves me, loves me not."
Remember picking the daisy petals and wondering?

Illustrating Principle II

Throughout the rest of the book, we will be applying this principle to foods and eating habits. We will show the importance of eating foods before they have had their natural nutrients processed away. In this chapter, however, I will illustrate the principle by applying it more broadly, showing that adhering to God's rules applies not only to what we swallow, but also to nondietary issues as well.

Laws Concerning Good Hygiene

An unusual subject about which God was very specific was regarding women and their menstrual cycle. In Leviticus 18:19, He commanded:

> *Do not approach a woman to have sexual relations during the uncleanness of her monthly period.*

Modern research has discovered

"My Daddy would beat me if I didn't steal and bring home money every night."

I couldn't believe my ears. This young child was actually expressing surprise upon hearing the Ten Commandments. I kept thinking he had misunderstood me or was kidding, but he wasn't. He had never heard of them.

Whether out of ignorance, rebellion or the theory that God's laws "no longer apply," humans often choose to go in a direction opposite from what God wants us to go.

> *Although they claimed to be wise, they became fools* (Rom. 1:22)

Many people, however, know better. This brings us to Principle II in our search for biblical patterns of eating:

> *As much as possible, eat foods as they were created—before they are changed or converted into something humans think are better.*

To underscore this rule, a related application is found in Proverbs 16:25:

> *There is a way that seems right to a man, but in the end it leads to death.*

"He loves me, he loves me not." Remember picking the daisy petals and wondering?

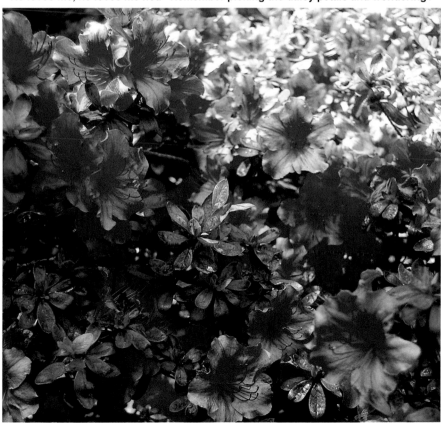

that a woman is much more susceptible to all infections during her period. These infections might be in the form of toxic shock syndrome, AIDS, yeast and fungi. Both sexual partners are more likely to be infected with the other's pathological germs during menstruation.

God's laws concerning hygiene were given to protect individuals and nations. Why would we want to change them? To do so is to violate Principle II.

God also said:

Designate a place outside the camp where you can go to relieve yourself (Deut. 23:12).

It seems logical to us today that keeping our living areas clean of urine and feces helps prevent disease. Science didn't discover this principle until relatively recently. God allowed His people to discover it by revelation. He wanted to protect them—and us—so He gave them very specific instructions. Through the ages, Jews who followed these rules were spared some of the major plagues and epidemics.

In the past, I have seen raw sewage in the streets of many countries I have visited. Perhaps many of our worldwide catastrophes could be prevented by following a simple rule written long ago.

Other Defilements

In Leviticus 20, we find both moral and dietary defilements. These include:

1. Sacrificing your children;
2. Turning to mediums or spiritualists;
3. Cursing one's parents;
4. Having sex with another man's wife;
5. Having sex with a family member other than your spouse;
6. Having sex with an animal;
7. Having sex with someone of your own gender;
8. Consulting with or acting as a medium or "familiar spirit";
9. Eating "unclean" flesh.

Isn't it interesting that God condemns unholy sexual relationships and eating unclean meats in the same chapter? Obviously, these forbidden

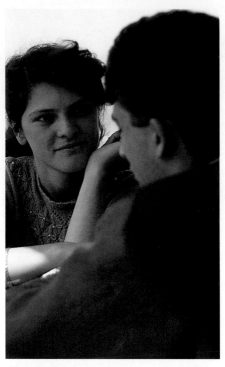

God demands pure sexual relationships.

items have both moral and physical implications.[1]

Sexual Defilements

Incest. The Lord said to Moses concerning incest:

"No one is to approach any close relative to have sexual relations. I am the Lord" (Lev. 18:6).

He concluded such commandments by saying,

"Do not defile yourselves in any of these ways, because this is how the nations that I am going to drive out before you became defiled" (v. 24).

This was the first time in history that siblings were not allowed to marry. Certainly brothers and sisters married in Adam and Eve's family—after the Fall. Siblings and family members continued to marry after the tower of Babel incident recorded in Genesis 11.[2] This widely accepted pattern of intermarriage within families explains the genetic development of the world's various races.[3]

Because of the curse, people's potential for harmful mutations has gradually increased, requiring the command that relatives not marry. If we ignore God's law about this issue, the results are harmful to the development of healthy genes. In other

words, it is a disaster for those groups that practice it.

An angry and vengeful God? The Author of this law must have been compassionate to be stern enough to help us avoid birth defects.

Adultery. God's Word is clear about the high price of sexual indiscretion. Under Old Testament law,

"If a man commits adultery with another man's wife—...both the adulterer and the adulteress must be put to death" (Lev. 20:10).

In the New Testament, however, we see a picture of Jesus pardoning the harlot caught in adultery just before the crowd is about to stone her, according to Mosaic law (see John 8:7). Thus, Jesus asserts His authority over Mosaic law—on the one hand affirming its essential aspects, and on the other bringing a new awareness of the role of mercy and grace. By no means, however, did Jesus condone adultery. On the contrary, He said:

"Anyone who looks at a woman lustfully has already committed adultery with her in his heart" (Matt. 5:28).

Jesus was teaching the Jews that the law is more than commands and ordinances—living right is an issue of the heart, including the mind, soul and body. Though we no longer stone adulterers, nonetheless, the consequences are grave for the body, mind and soul when this sinful act is committed.

For example, the syphilis epidemic that ravaged Europe during the 1600s resulted in the deaths of 50 percent of the population in some cities. One group, however, the Puritans, were protected from this scourge by enforcing strict standards against adultery.

The Consequences of Sexual Disobedience

Principle II has particular relevance when we consider some of the more popular ways many modern people ignore or pervert God's laws regarding sexuality.

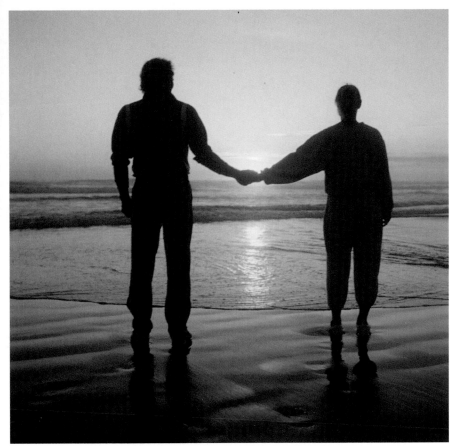

Many of the "AIDS awareness" campaigns emphasize "safe sex."

AIDS

Returning to Leviticus 18, God also said:

> *"Do not have sexual relations with an animal and defile yourself with it. A woman must not present herself to an animal to have sexual relations with it; that is a perversion"* (v. 23).

Peter Lewin, an epidemiologist from Toronto, believes that the AIDS virus was introduced to humans by this terrible "perversion."[4] Although the HIV virus is present in sheep, monkeys, pigs and cats, the animals themselves usually remain without symptoms[5]—transmission to humans occurs by eating the animal's flesh or by bestiality.[6]

Both eating unclean animals and having sexual relations with them are defilements listed in Leviticus 20, and are considered abominations punishable by exclusion or death. Was God cruel to punish these ancient peoples for engaging in bestiality or would He have been crueler to let this kind of activity go unchecked, leading to the possible deaths of millions?

AIDS and Homosexuality

God's law also speaks directly to the abomination of same-gender sex:

> *"Do not lie with a man as one lies with a woman; that is detestable"* (Lev. 18:22).
> *"If a man lies with a man as one lies with a woman, both of them have done what is detestable"* (20:13).

In the New Testament, the apostle Paul spoke of both men and women who had disobeyed this law:

> *Because of this, God gave them over to shameful lusts. Even their women exchanged natural relations for unnatural ones. In the same way the men also abandoned natural relations with women and were inflamed with lust for one another. Men committed indecent acts with other men* (Rom. 1:26,27).

Before 1987, all human HIV infections in Taiwan were passed through homosexual contacts.[7] This pattern has been repeated in every country where the routes of HIV transmissions have been studied.

What about those news reports that some researchers have decided homosexuality is inherited, or at least connected in some way to a person's genetic makeup? The *Atlantic Monthly* featured a long article written by a professing homosexual. After reviewing many such claims, the author concluded that no good evidence substantiated a genetic cause for homosexuality.[8] I often wonder: *Would a loving Creator design such a trait?*

The genetic link really does not make sense to me because natural selection teaches that the "trait" would be lost quickly because no offspring are produced to pass it on to succeeding generations. Also, this "trait" rapidly increases the death rate.

Dr. William Johnson, a secular sexual researcher of Masters and Johnson fame, reported a 70 percent reversal of the homosexual lifestyle when counseling therapy was used.[9] This was done without any gene therapy (i.e., changing a person's genetic makeup). The homosexual lifestyle is a confusing and real problem, but I believe the genetic origin of homosexuality theory has little credibility.

Safe(???) Sex

As you know, many of the "AIDS awareness" campaigns emphasize "safe sex," usually meaning the use of condoms when engaging in extramarital or same-sex activity. Let's look at the following facts:

1. In promiscuous sex, even with condoms, the infection rate is 100 percent with the human papilloma virus (HPV).[10] Some experts believe that HPV virus may cause infections, warts and eventually cancer of the cervix and penis.[11] In 1991, 46 percent of University of California coeds tested positive for HPV.[12] This condyloma-HPV virus has no cure.

2. Even with condoms, studies have shown a 30 percent infection rate in women whose spouse had HIV.[13] The condom apparently irritates the vagina, making it more susceptible to the infection. The infection rate of HIV from husbands to wives is only 3 percent when condoms are not used.[14]

The male who has HIV is more

likely to pass the disease to the female during her period. Conversely, the female who has HIV is more likely to pass the disease during the female's menstrual flow.[15] (See Lev. 18:19.)

3. Pregnancy occurs in 12 percent of couples who use a condom for protection.[16]

4. According to a review of the HIV virus by Dr. Lorraine Day, the virus is present in all the body fluids of an infected person. It can be cultured from sneezes that are up to 20 inches away. It stays alive in air, water and dry surfaces. It is not necessarily killed by antiseptic solutions such as alcohol.[17]

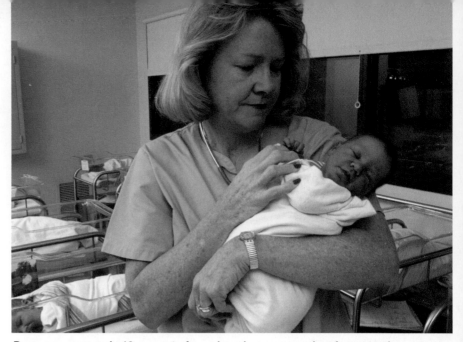

Pregnancy occurs in 12 percent of couples who use a condom for protection.

The "Judgment" of AIDS

Does God "judge" people who violate His moral laws by "giving" them AIDS? Or are such diseases simply the consequence of breaking His laws—similar to disobeying God's law of gravity?

Some confused Christians might claim that God singles out homosexuals for His special wrath, but I disagree. I think it is clear from the Scriptures that a kind of judgment for disobeying God's laws is built into Creation—for *anyone* who is disobedient (regardless of sexual orientation).

This is no more the work of a vengeful God than when a child is struck when walking into the path of an oncoming car. It is a part of the way a fallen world works.

Paul spoke of this in the same way immediately after denouncing homosexuality:

Men committed indecent acts with other men, and received in themselves the due penalty for their perversion (Rom 1:27).

God is not trying to limit sexual pleasure, but to enhance it. More than 26 highly contagious diseases are passed through homosexual activity. Once again, a loving Creator cared for us enough to reveal His law against this behavior, and warned that it would have tragic results.

The Mechanism Explained

Bear with me here so I can explain at least in part why God forbids homosexual activity.

Sperm are designed to swim and penetrate. The lining of the vagina is very tough, and is designed to withstand the severe trauma during childbirth. Neither viruses, bacteria nor sperm can penetrate the lining of the vagina, and it is difficult for viruses to penetrate the vaginal wall. Healthy sperm, however, can easily swim through the birth canal and into the uterus or oviduct to penetrate an ovum, starting a new life.

In contrast, the lining of the rectum is very fragile. Sperm placed in the rectum easily penetrate the mucosa and temporarily shut down the immune system, making the victim susceptible to infections. Thus, having a compromised immune system, any infection or latent cancer cells are poorly controlled. The consequences are often fatal.

Defilement and a Loving/Judging God

The Bible discusses sexual practices such as homosexuality in the context of "defilement" (e.g., Lev. 20). Laws against defilement were not issued from an angry God who wants to limit our pleasure, but from a Designer who loves us and knows what lifestyles are best for us.

This does not mean, however, that God is a pushover when people deliberately disobey Him.

In Leviticus 18:24 God said:

Do not defile yourselves in any of these ways, because this is how the nations that I am going to drive out before you became defiled.

God went on to say:

Even the land was defiled; so I punished it for its sin, and the land vomited out its inhabitants...for all these things were done by the people who lived in the land before you, and the land became defiled. And if you defile the land, it will vomit you out as it vomited out the nations that were before you (vv. 25,27,28).

Just in case you were speed-reading and missed it, this passage says twice that the land will vomit out its inhabitants if they defile themselves with illicit sexuality. Researching and writing this section has been nauseating to me, just as defilement apparently nauseates God. Furthermore, I feel uneasy as I consider the behavior that is becoming "accepted" in our society. Will God also drive us from the land? Is He loving or angry to place such stiff penalties on those who defile themselves?

In looking at a map of the world distribution of AIDS, it is essentially

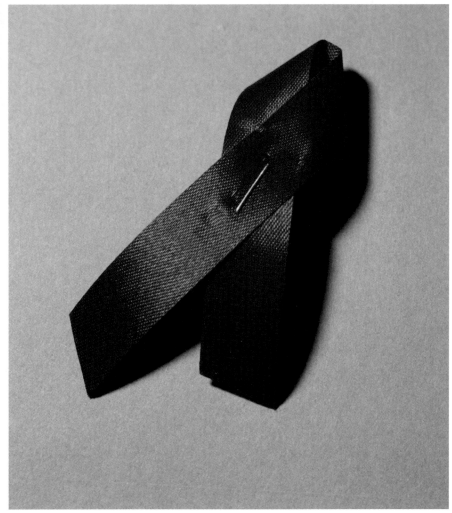

An AIDS ribbon. The virus presents little danger if we follow a healthful lifestyle.

end of the law, the moral and dietary laws of the Old Testament no longer applied, and therefore the Church was inconsistent in requiring people to follow these rules. He also believed that the God of the Old Testament was an angry, vengeful God, while the God of the New Testament was loving and gracious.

The radio preacher's approach was interesting to me because his logic paralleled my earlier logic, before my diet and lifestyle changes helped me overcome the worst effects of diabetes. He concluded, as I had, that the Old Testament was no longer pertinent. Its laws were outdated. We are under grace! So let us rid ourselves of these sexual and dietary religious restraints.

The homosexual preacher said that a loving God would not make such strict statements as, "Do not lie with a man as one lies with a woman; that is detestable" (Lev. 18:22). Neither would he exact such severe punishments as cutting off homosexuals from the rest of the people (see v. 29).

So this minister concluded that people were being cheated of many pleasures by these Old Testament moral standards.

Of course, he conveniently ignored the fact that the same standards are taught in the New Covenant. As we have seen, the apostle Paul charged that ungodly and lustful "men also abandoned natural relations with women and were inflamed with lust for one another" (Rom. 1:27).

Paul also asked, "Do you not know that your body is a temple of the Holy Spirit, who is in you, whom you have received from God?...Therefore honor God with your body (1 Cor. 6:19,20).

When the minister cited Romans 10:4, which says that "Christ is the end of the law," he conveniently left out two important words. Paul actually said that Christ is the end of the law *for righteousness*. Including those words changes the homosexual minister's whole conclusion. Christ *ended* the works of the law *as a means of being justified for salvation or sanctification.* By shedding His blood, He became the fulfillment of the sacrificial law. He made it possible for every person who will come to Him in repentance and faith to appropriate His own righteousness.

nonexistent in certain areas. In Saudi Arabia, which has very few cases of AIDS, homosexuality is prohibited. China, where the Communist regime also bans homosexuality, did not discover its first case until 1991.[18] If we compare the low incidence of AIDS in China to the high incidence in the United States, it seems a short step to conclude that this deadly "plague" is behavior related.

Dr. G. T. Stewart, emeritus professor of public health at the University of Glasgow, and others are realizing that a person's lifestyle is what causes the disease, independent of the HIV virus.[19] He notes that many of the 38 diseases commonly found in AIDS patients are common to the homosexual lifestyle even when no HIV infection is present. In other words, it's the lifestyle, not some virus sent from God, that destroys the body's built-in, divinely designed means of protecting

itself. The virus itself presents little danger to us if we follow the healthful lifestyle outlined in Scripture and summarized in The Three Principles.

Wise parents, concerned about their child's safety, teach the child about the dangers of playing in traffic. Parents who also discipline the child who rebels and runs out into a busy street are demonstrating love, not cruelty. Playing with lifestyles that are against God's loving rules is also dangerous, and we cannot fairly charge God with cruelty when He disciplines us for disobeying laws that were given for our health.

Does Grace Cancel Reality?

I once heard a self-professed homosexual radio preacher try to justify his lifestyle by using Romans 10:4, which says that "Christ is the end of the law." He reasoned that because Jesus was the

Paul also wrote:

Shall we go on sinning, so that grace may increase? By no means! We died to sin; how can we live in it any longer? (6:1,2).

Let me state clearly that I believe a scriptural approach to homosexuality involves loving the homosexual, while hating the practice of homosexuality. In this respect, it is no different from other sins. When I am guilty, say, of willfully disobeying traffic laws, I would hope for Christians to love me, at the same time pointing out the error of my ways. I believe the Christian challenge is to deal in a similar way with homosexuals.

Hope, Health and the Christian Way

Arno Karlen, in writing about the history of plagues and epidemics, describes a world in which humans and nature are in conflict. He believes that nature uses microbes to destroy humans as world populations increase. It's a matter of the survival of the fittest. His assertion is that epidemics are nature's way of culling the weak. Karlen states:

The moral theme appeared early in the age of pandemics; It was encouraged by the fact that plagues paid dividends to Christianity.[20]

The author explains that during the Roman Empire people fled to Christianity because of its messages of hope and chastisement of wrongdoers. He then tries to assure his readers that the Romans' worship of food, drink, sex and self had nothing to do with the frequent epidemics they suffered.

I believe this view has led to an error in interpreting the causes of epidemics. The Christian message included definite standards of what was right and wrong. In addition to hope, another attraction to Christianity was health. Results have always been impressive when biblical standards for health and hygiene were followed.

Archeologists have noticed that during the Roman Empire, Roman cities and camps planned their sewage and cisterns in the center of their

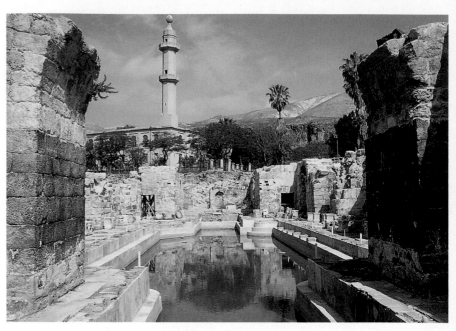

Roman baths, Israel. Roman townplanning made people vulnerable to epidemics.

compounds—allowing their water to be contaminated and leaving themselves vulnerable to seeping epidemics and plagues. In contrast, both Jewish and Muslim communities in many eras have been spared such tragedies simply by following the hygienic principles of water and waste commanded in their Scriptures.

Rome and other opponents of Christianity were offended by the protection early Christians seemed to enjoy from epidemics. Did jealousy regarding this apparent "favoritism," as well as the rapid spread of the faith around the world and the early Christians' refusal to pay homage to the gods of Rome, play together to make Rome want to persecute Christians?

A similar reaction can be seen by the opponents of the Jews during the "black plague" that killed millions during the Middle Ages. Many European Jews suffered great persecution because others noticed they were spared the disease. Actually, the mechanisms of protection were related to seeking pure water and separating themselves from their sewage—just as God commanded (see Deut. 23:12,13).

In contrast, many non-Jews let fecal material lie exposed in their streets and homes. They did not protect their water supplies, and they ate unclean foods. Millions of Jews and Christians also died needlessly when they

decided not to follow the biblical ordinances and commands. They supposed the cause of the plagues was "spontaneous generation"—an evil springing from nothing.

Of course, many of the common people didn't have access to the Scriptures during the Middle Ages. Then, in the nineteenth century, Louis Pasteur designed experiments negating the possibility of spontaneous generation. He developed the germ theory, vaccines and sterilization techniques, and the more he learned scientifically, the greater his faith became in the supernatural God of the Bible. His discoveries began to check some of the terrible epidemics.

This kind of evidence shows how biblical principles have a direct bearing on human health and hope. No one has to "count petals" to know that God loves us, regardless of our sinful state. The standards He has set for healthy living are a sign of this great love.

5. Principle III

Don't Let Any Food or Drink Become Your God

*We have said that food is the best medicine.
No food can be good medicine, too!*

If I put up the swing set and discover that too many pieces are left over, and that it is not balanced right, I might want to look at the directions!

My investigation into fasting as a means of healing diseases began in just that way. When I observed the lives of several people who are near and dear to me, it was clear they were out of balance.

Sue, a bright, cute nine-year-old, had severe dyslexia. Her loving and interested family had the means to take her to the best medical facilities in the country for evaluation. She was being tutored by a teacher who was an expert in learning problems.

At one point, Sue became ill with the flu and couldn't eat for several days. When the teacher returned, he found to his surprise that Sue could read! He remarked to the parents, "I don't know what you are doing but please don't quit. She is reading above her expected reading level."

Does this mean that rest, fever and fasting will correct dyslexia?

When Sue resumed her normal diet, her reading problems returned. Later, when she experimented and ate only unfamiliar foods, her reading skills improved. Further testing revealed that she was sensitive to sugar, corn, white flour, margarine, honey and several other frequently eaten foods. As you might suspect, the foods she liked best were the most offending.

Another observation I made was in my immediate family. We had a son who was hyperactive. Several kinds of therapy were unsatisfactory. Another plan included a three-day fast prior to treatment. Having never considered fasting before, we were a little scared and apprehensive. Rather than a water fast, we let our son eat only foods he had never eaten before—plums, kiwis, fish, cashews and so on.

We were absolutely astounded by the third day to see him being calm. We thought he was lethargic, but he was probably just acting normal. Many of his favorite foods stimulated him to extremes of activity and lack of concentration. Of course, it was hard—almost impossible—to keep him interested in eating certain foods instead of junk foods, so our troubles had not completely ended. Knowing some help might be available somewhere, however, was hopeful. We decided to investigate further into what happens when the body is deprived of certain foods. *What is fasting, anyway?* we wondered.

What Is a Fast?

According to *Grolier's Encyclopedia,* fasting is the following:

The practice of abstaining from food, either completely or partially, for a specified period. It is an ancient practice found in most religions of the world.

The normal fast is not eating food for a definite time period.

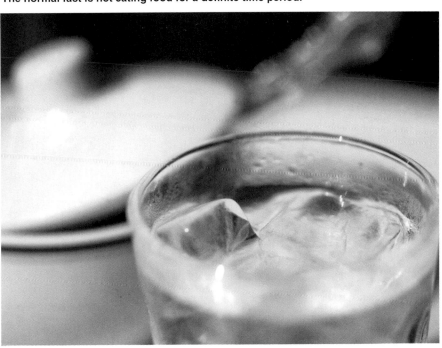

Traditionally, fasting has been a widely used form of asceticism, and a penitential practice observed for the purpose of purifying the person or atoning for sins and wrong-doing.

Most religions designate certain days or seasons as times of fasting for their adherents, such as Lent, Yom Kippur and Ramadan. Certain events in the lives of individual persons have been considered appropriate times for fasting, such as the day or night before a major personal commitment. The vigil of knighthood is a historical instance of this practice.

Prayer is supposed to accompany fasting. In this respect, fasting should be distinguished from abstinence.

History and Background

Hippocrates, the father of medicine, used fasting to combat disease 2,400 years ago. The ancient Ayurvedic healers of the Hindu religion prescribed fasting weekly for a healthy digestive system. Most nationalities, religions and languages have a tradition of fasting handed down from their ancestors.

Most secular historians speculate that fasting evolved from people living without food during troubled times. Eventually they learned to be without food because they were troubled. I think I know a better explanation.

The Chinese have fasted since their beginnings, which some scholars think was four generations after Noah's family lived. The earliest writings in the Chinese language are inscribed on bones and pottery—dated 2000 B.C. These writings include stories of a seven-day Creation, the Fall of humans from their favored place in a garden, a great flood and many other accounts also recorded in Genesis. Similar flood stories are found in more than 200 ancient languages, including several Native American accounts.

The fact that fasting is found in many languages would indicate that this practice occurred before the Tower of Babel incident. The story is history: The ruins of the tower can be seen in present-day Iraq. The people of Babel were the descendants of Noah. The practice of fasting may have been handed down through Noah's offspring. Did Noah, in turn, receive the tradition from the very week of Creation itself, when God "rested" on the seventh day? Could it be that Sabbath rest was designed for the digestive system as well as for a religious observance?

Four Kinds of Fasting

1. The *normal fast* is not eating food for a definite time period. The duration can be one day, as noted in Judges 20:26:

> Then the Israelites, all the people, went up to Bethel, and there they sat weeping before the Lord. They fasted that day until evening and presented burnt offerings and fellowship offerings to the Lord.

Biblical fasts were also observed for three days, one week, one month and as long as 40 days. Extreme care should be taken with longer fasts, and medical advice from a physician is necessary.

Advice from a physician is necessary for longer fasts.

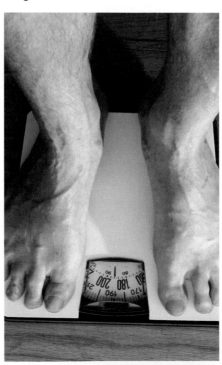

2. The *absolute fast* is not ingesting food or water, and should be short. Moses' 40-day fast would kill anyone who does not have supernatural intervention. Be sure to test the spirit that tries to talk you into a 40-day fast without water, because normally it is a physical impossibility.

3. The *partial fast* includes omitting one meal a day, or omitting certain foods for a specific time period. Eating only fresh vegetables for several days is a good partial fast. John Wesley ate only bread (whole grain) and drank water for many days. Elijah fasted (partially) twice. John the Baptist and Daniel along with his three friends are other examples of partial fasts. People who have hypoglycemia or other diseases could benefit from this kind of fast.

4. A *rotational fast* involves avoiding certain foods periodically. For example, food families such as grains are eaten only every fourth day. Three days of fasting without grains of any kind may be followed by one day of eating grains. The various food families are rotated so that some food is available each day.

Benefits of Fasting

From the very beginning, before the Fall of humans, our bodies were designed to take periodic rests from food. The seventh day was designed for rest, and the digestive system needs rest just as much as does the body.

Healing and Rest

One of the main benefits of a night's sleep includes rest for the digestive system. It is no accident that in English the first meal of the day is named "break-fast." A 12- to 14-hour fast can also be beneficial for the system. One school of thought once taught that many health benefits are gained by skipping the traditional breakfast and waiting until noon or later to eat. (Many like to do this now, but receive criticism from Mom, medicine and other people. Are you too afraid of them to miss a meal?)

We know that foods (nutrients) are necessary for health. Because of this

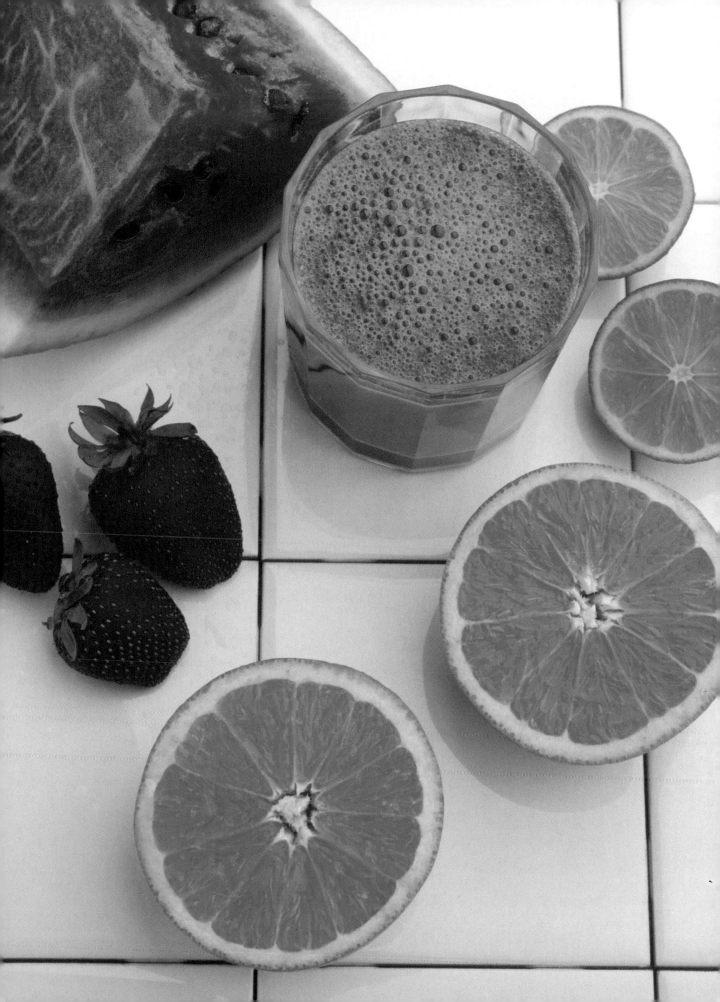

necessity it was once hard for me to recommend fasting. My logic was that if eating is healthful, not eating was harmful. I now realize that this logic was faulty. You fast, whether you call it that or not, when you don't eat from 9:00 P.M. until 6:00 A.M. Extending this fast for a reasonable time won't harm you either.

Your body was designed to respond to sickness in a certain way. Fever, fasting and rest are part of the design! Do you remember the last time you were sick? Did you want to eat? Did you want to party? No! You had a temperature, could not keep any food down and only wanted to crawl into your bed and be left alone.

Why do we work so hard to lower our temperatures? Fever causes us to ache and to want to lie down. We fight going to bed because we are motivated by several excuses. "Strong people don't quit!" and "They can't work without me!" (Of course fever as high as 106 degrees can cause death or brain damage, and should be treated quickly. Body temperature should be kept under 104 degrees.) Rest, fever and fasting seem to be part of the design to shorten viral infections.

Have you heard that you can "sweat off a cold"? It sounds bizarre, but if the work or exercise causes your body to warm up it might help. Researchers have also discovered that many harmful viruses do not multiply at temperatures much more than 100 degrees. Fever is also reported to increase the mobility of the white blood cells, which destroy bacteria and viruses. Researchers are now heating the blood of AIDS patients to reduce viral counts, hoping to gain remissions.

The body is designed to heal itself at the cellular level. The biochemical mechanisms of the cell are billions of times more complex than the precise mechanisms that cause the universe to function. These processes utilize proteins, carbohydrates and fats to gain calories and nutrients for untold other reactions. Each reaction also produces waste products. The cells have ways to clear this waste, but apparently they can become overloaded. Fasting helps unclog the system, and also eliminates poison from it. The cell uses periods of rest to process and

eliminate waste or other toxins. Modern research, ancient healers and more importantly the Word of the body's Designer—God—indicate that one benefit of fasting is healing.

In Isaiah 58:8, God took Israel to task for abusing the fast. He said that if they really fasted according to His will, "Then your light will break forth like the dawn, and your healing will quickly appear."

In the nineteenth century, Dr. Isaac Jennings learned to prescribe rest, fasting and fresh pure water as a treatment for fever—instead of the bloodletting, heat and water deprivation that were conventional medicine's practices at the time.[1]

Dr. Jennings developed a reputation for reversing many chronic illnesses. He prescribed a variety of colored pills, powders and water, while withholding food for various periods of time (partial fasting). His success was so phenomenal that Yale University conferred an honorary degree upon him.

When Dr. Jennings revealed that his pills and powders were small, stained fragments of bread, his acclaim dwindled. He had discovered the placebo effect, but had he also rediscovered the far-encompassing benefits of fasting?

Exercise helps warm the body.

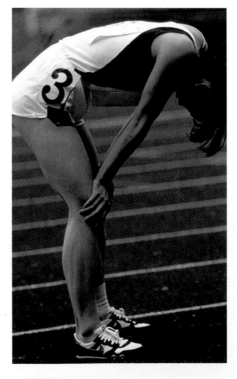

Fasting and Cancer Research

Research by Dr. George Thampy, a biochemist at the University of Indiana, on 60 healthy subjects who participated in a three-week fast revealed interesting results: (1) significant lowering of cholesterol; (2) lowering of blood pressure; (3) relief from arthritis; (4) loss of body mass and weight (as much as 40 pounds during the three-week fast).[2]

Those subjects who broke the fast and maintained a Genesis 1:29 (vegetarian) diet did not regain much weight even one month after breaking the fast. Those subjects who abruptly switched to a normal diet regained significant weight (as much as 15 pounds) during the first week of refeeding.

Currently Thampy is "chasing" a certain factor that is known to kill tumor cells. This factor is absent in tumor patients, and may be elevated in fasting subjects.

Fasting has also been shown to be an effective treatment for rheumatoid arthritis, and can reduce joint pains, swelling and morning stiffness in just a few days. In one experiment, 27 rheumatoid arthritis patients stayed on a Genesis 1:29 diet—basically a vegetarian diet—and showed remarkable improvement. Another group of patients in the same test did not stick to the partial fast and suffered relapses.[3]

Fasting and Mental Health

Mental benefits of fasting include a calming effect, the ability to focus on priorities and a generalized improvement in mental functioning.

Don't expect mental miracles on your first fast. Addiction and withdrawal symptoms (irritability, anger, headaches and so on) could override any first-time benefits. Examples of fasting's positive effect on the mind, however, are even more striking.

A Kansas couple I know, both of them physicians, had an autistic son. They discovered fasting when the boy was 12 years old. After the son's three-day fast, he began to respond to them for the first time in his life. Through testing it was learned he had an enzyme deficiency that made him sensitive to certain foods. After a general fast of a few days, a rotational fast was used to keep from over-

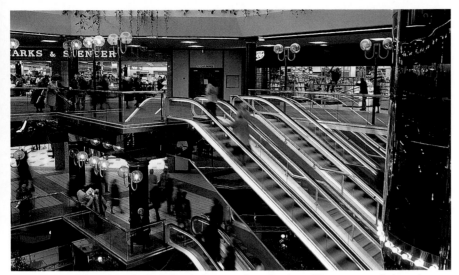

Society is addicted to alcohol, food, drugs, education, wealth, power and shopping.

whelming the son's enzyme system. At age 18 the boy was reading and showing great improvement, according to his parents.

The symptoms of many other neurological disorders, such as hyperactivity, dyslexia, incorrigible delinquency, schizophrenia and depression, apparently have cleared temporarily during short fasts. These syndromes are usually blamed on early childhood/parental relationships; but what if they are more closely related to diet?

The psychoanalysts who followed Sigmund Freud's theory for years did so with almost cultlike devotion. Freud is still revered as the father of psychiatry. Freud's guilt-producing theory about the subconscious id, ego and superego was primarily accepted because academia was using a new definition for science that excluded the supernatural. A cocaine user himself, Freud formulated his theory and gained his fame by treating patients with cocaine. The patients reported wonderful results, but he produced a bizarre theory. "There is a way that seems right to a man, but in the end it leads to death" (Prov. 14:12).

In the strictest definition, Freud's methods became a religion; but since his day, most of these psychological diseases have been shown to have organic causes. Some of the symptoms of these mental illnesses have reportedly disappeared after receiving kidney dialysis, which filters toxic products from the blood. These products rebuild rapidly, and within a few hours the symptoms may return.

Could the toxins come from incompletely metabolized foods, or an accumulation of waste products? Can chemicals or drugs cause bizarre symptoms? Sure!

The mind is a precious thing. Fasting can give the body time to clear itself of toxic products. Eating things designed for food in their purest form could be great for the mind, just as it has been shown to maintain our joints, our weight and our immune system.

Dr. Yuri Nikolayave, a psychiatrist at the University of Moscow, treated schizophrenics with water fasts for 25 to 30 days. This was followed by eating foods in their purest forms for 30 days. Seventy percent of his patients remained free from symptoms for the duration of the 6-year study.[4] In patients who have these advanced illnesses, profound biochemical changes do occur during the fast.

Allan Cott, an M.D. at New York University, has used this fasting treatment on 28 schizophrenic patients. He reported a 60 percent recovery rate from this dreaded illness.[5]

For many similar cases, read *Brain Allergies* by Dr. William Philpott, who is a neuropsychiatrist. He treated food reactions by withdrawal of the offending foods for three months. Then he rotated meals by food families every four days. Dr. Philpott uses this treatment for all kinds of physical and psychological problems, including arthritis, and has surprising success.[6]

The rotation diet is complex and difficult, even for highly motivated patients. It appears to me that a yoke of bondage to foods and chemicals is more easily broken by frequent periods of abstinence (fasting). A three-month withdrawal of the offending food is the equivalent of a fast from that food.

Pediatricians, cardiologists, internists and many other specialists use this form of unconventional treatment for many ailments and have outstanding results, but supervision is a necessity.

Don't expect medical or mental miracles on your first fast.

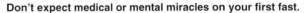

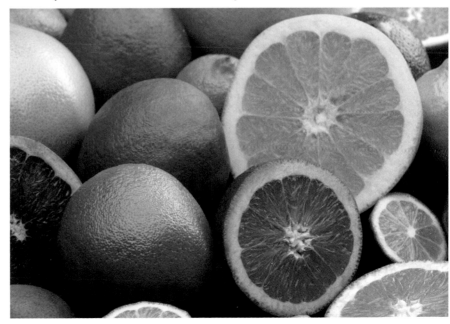

Food Addictions

It is possible to make any item of food your god by becoming addicted to it. Anything that becomes an addiction displaces God from His rightful throne in our lives. "Jeshurun (Israel) grew fat and kicked; filled with food, he became heavy and sleek. He abandoned the God who made him" (Deut. 32:15).

In his classic devotional work, *My Utmost for His Highest*, Oswald Chambers wrote: "Make it a habit to have no habits." He emphasized that Christ is your Lord, which means "boss." If you are Christ's slave, even your good habits may keep you from serving Him. Eating is a necessary habit some have elevated to the realm of worship. Don't let any chemical, food or drink become your god.

On the same principle, don't become addicted to fasting either. Don't be deceived into believing that you should not eat healthfully. You need many nutrients at frequent intervals. Occasional fasting is the exception to the rule of eating.

Our society is addicted to alcohol, sports, food, drugs, education, wealth, power, work, relationships, nicotine, gambling, shopping and so on. According to some researchers, more than 10 million people in the United States alone are negatively affected by the use of some toxic substance.[7] According to *The Kellogg Report*:

As peculiarly contemporary illnesses, they are caused by affluent overloads of once rare substances, from nicotine to sugar to cocaine, that now flood our society.[8]

Many things to which we are addicted are good in themselves. Food, sex, money and work are all wonderful blessings if used by the guidelines for their design. In my experience, these guidelines are best found in Scripture. Diet, however, is usually affected negatively by addictions. We have only to note the harmful effects of alcohol, eating disorders, drugs and smoking. Because these addictions cause us to eat improperly, the solution involves

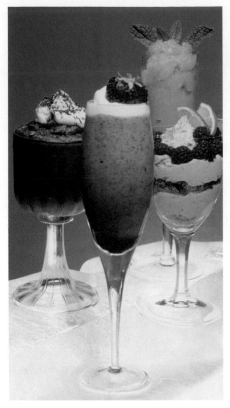

It is possible to make any item of food your god by becoming addicted to it.

proper food intake, as well as proper emotions. Both eating and emotions are affected positively by proper fasting.

Other addictions that affect us negatively include sugar, fat and caffeine. These substances not only cause us to neglect essential nutrients, but they also make the body lose its ability to digest, absorb and utilize the nutrients it needs. If addictions were broken or prevented by fasting, nutrients designed for our cells could be digested, absorbed and utilized. When fasting is combined with eating the things created for food, "then your healing will . . . appear" (Isa. 58:8).

Preventing health problems is much easier than recovering from health problems. In general, fasting will prevent addiction to foods.

Humans have imperfect enzyme systems (remember that the Fall of humans placed limitations on the body: "Cursed are you" [Gen. 3:14]). Each person's "fallen" enzyme system is unique. This is why one person may be sensitive to milk and the next person can consume large amounts without any problems. One person could spend a lifetime trying to evaluate how each particular food affects his or her body.

Regular intervals of fasting appear to be a better way of protecting ourselves from a deficient or an imperfect enzyme system. Fasting prevents low levels of enzymes from being overwhelmed by gluttony or overconsumption. Perhaps fasting is a way to counter this aspect of the Fall—a way designed from the beginning when our Creator created a day for rest.

It is said that the brain wants the very substance that is doing it the most harm. In truth, we cannot trust our own brains to want what is best for us. That is another reason we need food standards such as those presented in Scripture. The brain tells us it wants more sugar, fat and other luxuries found in what is popularly called "fast food." The brain likes this food, but if too much is consumed, the body begins to rebel with sickness and/or poor health, and if the cycle is constantly repeated, gluttony and addiction begin to form. Proverbs 23 warns:

When you sit to dine with a ruler, note well what is before you, and put a knife to your throat if you are given to gluttony. Do not crave his delicacies, for that food is deceptive (vv. 1-3).

Dr. Beasley compares the behavior of addicted persons to a burning building:

Every cell of (the body) is gradually being consumed and destroyed by the effects of their addiction or compulsion. Without a recovered body, neither the mind nor the spirit can reach its full potential.[9]

Dr. Richard Weindruch of the University of California in Los Angeles reported that fasting mice frequently lived longer and had significantly fewer diseases than mice that were allowed to eat anytime they wanted.[10]

An addiction to foods such as sugar, salt, fat or caffeine will not be cleared by a 24-hour period of abstinence. Often food addictions require from three weeks to three months of abstinence to clear the system from the offending food. Frequent short periods of abstinence may help eventually to clear bondage to food.

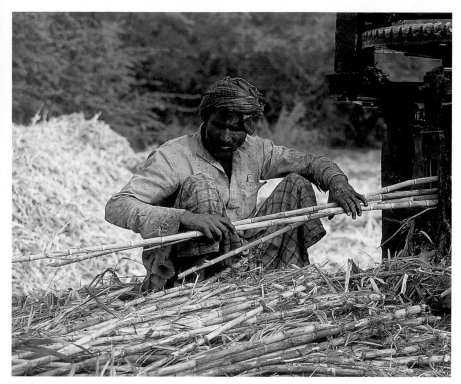

An Indian farmer making sugar from cane. Many people are addicted to sugar.

What to Expect, How to Start

Three days before you start your fast, eat only things God created for food, and in the purest, most natural form possible—before basic nutrients have been processed from the foods. Drinking pure water during a fast is wise.

On the first day of a fast, I recommend drinking only water and juice, and no sweeteners. This helps counteract hypoglycemic symptoms many people experience during their first fast. The number of symptoms and their severity may depend on the food addictions you have accumulated. Most symptoms will be mild, consisting of a headache, weakness or irritability. Other symptoms may include bad breath, frequent urination, sleeplessness or a sensation of coolness.

If you feel sick, eat. You do not get extra "macho" points by making yourself suffer. Then try to fast again in a few days, trying to extend the duration of your fast a little longer.

Try stretching the hours by eating lunch, then skipping supper. You will be sleeping during the toughest time of the fast. Then you can "break fast" with praise for the food God has designed for you. Before long you will be able to go for 24 hours with water or juice only. You will feel great

On the first day of a fast drink only water and juice.

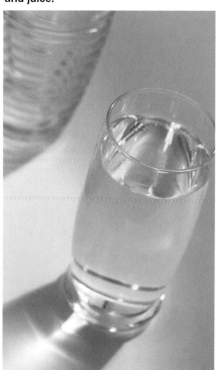

throughout most of your fast! Fasting this way once or even twice a week may be a great benefit for you. Later you can extend the fast to three days every month or two. Study books about fasting, such as *Fasting for Spiritual Breakthrough* by Elmer Towns (Regal Books, 1996). Let God direct you for longer fasts. You will not be the first to complete a long fast.

For partial fasts, you may want Day 1 to consist of juices, raw fruits and vegetables, and soups.

On Day 2, you could add whole-grain breads, nuts and cooked vegetables and legumes.

Take note of any symptoms that develop as you gradually replace your fast with food. If you develop symptoms after adding certain food, try avoiding it for several months.

After fasting, make meats only an occasional or celebrative food.

Most people who rely heavily on fasting for health purposes recommend an occasional weekend fast or even a weeklong fast. I can assure you that if you're healthy, this kind of fasting won't be harmful to you. Many people have completed fasts of up to 40 days without harming themselves; many have recovered from various maladies during times of fasting.

Supplementing your fast with freshly squeezed juices and broths may be helpful. Even a partial fast with vegetables may reduce symptoms. Seek medical or nutritional advice for your specific problems.

Fasting is not a competitive sport. You do not have to set any records. Your body does not get healthier if you out-fast your friend or opponent. Don't sulk if your spouse "out-fasts" you. God does not give you more pleasure or a special crown for suffering more than anyone else. There is no scorecard!

Protesters in Ireland who have refused food showed no ill effects until genuine hunger developed. When real hunger develops, the body is beginning to deteriorate and food is needed. Some Irish protesters who were healthy after 50 days of partial fasting died within two weeks after the onset of real hunger.

Avoid all teas, coffee (i.e., caffeine), sodas (i.e., sugar) during a fast.

Distilled or pure water and freshly squeezed juice are preferred. Remember also Jesus' counsel:

"When you fast, do not look somber as the hypocrites do, for they disfigure their faces to show men they are fasting. I tell you the truth, they have received their reward in full. But when you fast, put oil on your head and wash your face" (Matt. 6:16,17).

Jesus assumed we would pray, give alms, fast and forgive. His teachings assumed that all believers practiced these disciplines. For Him to give instruction about these practices to the believers was like discussing breathing, sleeping or eating, which were all assumed to be a part of a normal person's life.

The rewards of observing a fast include spiritual, mental and physical benefits. I believe that fasting is a valuable way to experience the Divine Design for total health.

Although the Bible and valid research indicates fasting is beneficial, it will still be hard to fast because of peer pressure and counsel from our families and medical advisors. Weight loss programs as well teach you to eat every meal. If we need three meals a day, does that mean every day? Are three meals a day needed? Who said?

Is that really healthful? (We often forget that three square meals can make us round!). Which is the healthier—fasting or never missing a meal? Proceed carefully and with a plan.[11]

Why do so many of us find fasting difficult?

The Root of Our Problem

Our major problem in fasting is the same as in other practices we know are good and wholesome, but that we have difficulty doing. It is both a time problem and a spiritual problem. We are too busy—not only to fast, but also to study God's Word, to engage in good works, to reflect on God's will for us, our community, church, family and nation. We are too busy to use the tools for the redeemed that would allow us to flourish.

Think about this, however: fasting could give you at least three extra hours a day. Consider all the time you spend in food preparation, in eating— and in postmeal bloated drowsiness! More time is also spent in deciding where, what, when, why and how we are going to eat.

Does history reveal that godly people were preoccupied with eating? On the contrary; many heroes and heroines of the faith spent time fasting—people such as Moses, David, Nehemiah, Esther, Daniel, Elijah, Hannah, Jesus, Paul, John and his disciples, and Anna.

Furthermore, many leaders God has used throughout history have practiced fasting, including Luther, Calvin, Wesley and Knox. Reading about their lives and work makes it evident that fasting was vital both to their relationship with their Creator and to their leadership and influence.

Recently Dr. Bill Bright of Campus Crusade for Christ asked 300 Christian leaders to join him in Orlando, Florida, to fast and pray. Surprisingly, 600 people from various organizations came and fasted with him for three days! Books such as Dr. Bright's *The Coming Revival* and Arthur Wallis's *The Chosen Fast* document the movement of the Holy Spirit on people of our time when they practice the discipline of fasting.

Perhaps fasting will bring revival to our land. I would like to be a part of it—wouldn't you?

PART 3

DINNER ACCORDING TO THE DIVINE DESIGN

*Here's a simple menu
showing the agreement
between modern research
and Divine Design.*

6. Going with the Grain (and Nuts, too)

Are grains and seeds too good to be true?
They are a part of God's wise design.

It's Monday morning, the day of new beginnings. My technicians at the hospital greet me cheerfully holding a box of glazed doughnuts, and ask innocently, "Dr. Russell, these are OK to eat, aren't they?"

My standard reply is, "Sure, if you want naked calories from lard, sugar and more sugar, and white flour."

I'm sure they're thinking, *Does that mean it's OK or not? Doesn't he like* anything? *What does he eat, anyhow?*

Why not train ourselves to like *everything* God made for our good—including the grain as He created it—whole—instead of refining and bleaching out its nutrients? Eating whole grains may be one of the most important factors in your return to good health.

Bread from God

At the beginning of our odyssey to health, someone told my wife and me that "Ezekiel bread" was a good and healthful bread.

What is Ezekiel bread? It originates from the days when God was instructing the prophet Ezekiel to demonstrate the siege that was to come upon the city of Jerusalem in punishment for the people's unfaithfulness. Ezekiel was to lie on his left side and then on his right side for 390 days each, apparently to show how helpless and paralyzed the city would be in front of its enemies.

To sustain the prophet's life during these long days, God told Ezekiel:

Take thou also unto thee wheat, and barley, and beans, and lentiles, and millet, and fitches, and put them in one vessel, and make thee bread thereof (Ezek. 4:9, KJV).

My wife, who follows recipes carefully, had a vague notion of what "lentiles" (lentils) and millet were, but could not interpret "fitch." Our Webster's dictionary said a fitch was a polecat. Fortunately, we knew that polecats are unclean, so we didn't pursue one as an ingredient for bread. There had to be another definition.

A Bible dictionary and a more modern recipe for Ezekiel bread revealed that fitch is a form of rye. I had never been much of a fan of rye bread, but I was sure I preferred it more than I preferred skunk. We made the bread and it was good,

although it was a little heavier than we were used to eating. The ingredients included wheat, barley, pinto beans, soybeans, lentils and millet.

Apparently this kind of bread was good for the prophet Ezekiel. After lying around for more than a year, it is recorded that he got up and walked.

Ezekiel bread has been analyzed and eaten by many people through the years. It has the complete package of essentials for health. It can be bought either as flour or bread at some whole-food stores. Many people have used it during times of sickness and have given good reports, although I know of no research that documents its effects.

Grains and Seeds: Too Good to Be True?

Genesis 1:29 says that God gave us every seed for food. Seeds are fashioned into at least three forms: grains, beans (legumes) and nuts.

Seeds seem almost too good to be true. They reproduce themselves at rates of 100 to 1,000 times a year. They supply everything we need for food. If we choose to eat meat, it comes from animals whose flesh has been nourished by eating grain or seeds.

Genesis 1:29 says that God gave us every seed for food.

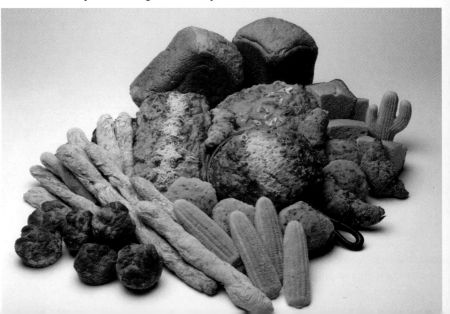

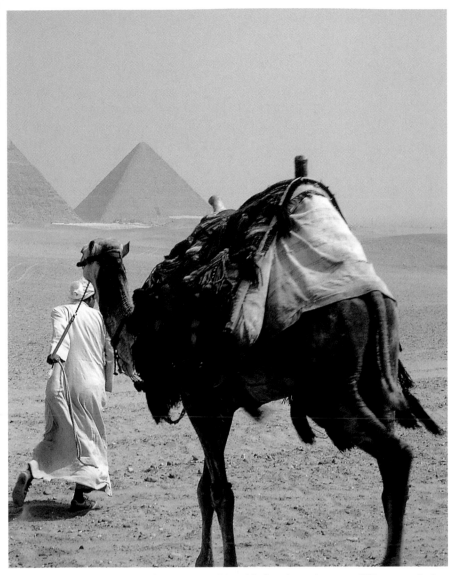

Wheat kernels found buried in the pyramids with the pharaohs can still be sprouted.

lysine? The fact is, we needed every ingredient from the first day of creation until now to survive and to reproduce.

4. In this complex world we need different seeds and grains for different nutrients, climates, altitudes and tastes. All the facts point to a Creator whose diverse designs included barley and buckwheat, corn and millet, oats, rice, rye, sorghum (milo), wheat, sesame and others. In addition, almost any seed can be used for grain.

More than 2,000 varieties of barley alone are available. Americans eat a lot of wheat, corn and rice, but in other countries millet is the staff of life.

People have always recognized the value of seeds. Not only has grain been used for food since the beginning, but it has also been used as money and a sign of wealth.

The Anatomy of a Design

The basic features of grain include the hull, the bran, the endosperm and the embryo. Each part performs an essential function. Although the nutrients found in each layer are vastly different, each layer of the grain-nut indicates that Someone had our good in mind when He created it.

Anatomy at Work

The *hull* (chaff) of a kernel of grain or seed is the part that is discarded or burned because it has no nutritional value. In addition, chaff is an irritant, causing the skin to itch. Ask anyone who has experienced a wheat harvest. The hull surrounds and protects the inner portions of the grain, preserving its overall nutritious value.

The *bran* is well designed into several layers. Its waxy outer coat (the *epicarp*) is another guard of both the nutrients and the life of the kernel within. This outer coat has a high cellulose content that is not a nutrient, but is the component that gives the kernel storage life and protects its ability to reproduce "after its kind."

Once this outer layer is penetrated, the nutrients start to deteriorate. As

A scientific examination of seeds indicates that they could not have developed by random chance. Their unique qualities point to the fact that they were designed by a benevolent Creator. Consider the following evidence:

1. A Designer would make grains available to all people everywhere. Grains can be easily grown from the Arctic in the Northern Hemisphere to the Antarctic in the Southern Hemisphere. Is it only an accident of evolution that they don't grow only in warm and wet climates?

2. A benevolent Designer would have designed grains to have good storage life. Farmers frequently store grains in elevators or on the ground until buyers can be found. In the pyramids of Egypt, kernels of wheat found buried with the pharaohs can still be sprouted 4,000 years later! What if this grain could only be stored one to five days? How would next year's crop be planted? Is it reasonable to suppose that a new seed would evolve in time to keep humans and animals alive? Preposterous!

3. If grains were made for humans and beasts, they would meet our needs. As it "happens," all our nutritional needs are met by seeds, including grains, nuts or legumes. What if only corn had evolved and we had no other grasses, grains or legumes containing the amino acid "lysine"? Without this single substance, humans and animals would not have survived. How could it have required many millions of years for corn to evolve into a pinto bean or a walnut, containing we progress inwardly toward the kernel of the grain, each layer has less cellulose but more vitamins, minerals, insoluble and soluble fiber, and proteins.

The proteins in a seed are of the highest quality and usefulness for us. Some are enzymes that are important in allowing us to properly digest the rest of the kernel. This design makes the grain's important nutrients more available to us.

The *endosperm* or starch part of the grain nourishes the embryo before the leaves have begun photosynthesis (the formation of carbohydrates by the action of light). The starch is stored in tiny packets separated from each other by gauze-thin membranes made of protein. These packets are like minute bundles of food that are released gradually—and in just the right sequence for the precise needs of the sprout until its roots and leaves can take control. Eventually the leaves and roots react with water, chlorophyll, sunlight and the carbon dioxide in the air to make carbohydrates (CHO).

The *embryo* or germ is shaped like a kidney or a bean (OK, like a kidney bean). In Deuteronomy 32:14 (KJV), Moses sang of how God had originally given man "the fat of kidneys of wheat" for food. Upon germination, the germ of a seed sprouts leaves and roots—which are one of the richest sources of vitamins B and E, and a rich source of the two essential fats and proteins. Although many gurus of medicine thought vitamin E was of no clinical importance until just a few years ago, God knew its value from the beginning.

Life by Design

Plants utilize the carbohydrates made by photosynthesis. The plant expels oxygen into the air as a waste product. And guess what—creation is designed so that animals need this oxygen: The carbohydrates manufactured by plants supply energy needs for the animals that eat the plants. The animals also need oxygen to metabolize the plants they eat. Animals emit carbon dioxide (CO_2) as a waste product, which in turn enriches the plants.

What if by chance the bran layer had the cellulose in the inner layers of the bran coating instead of its outer layers? The storage capacity would be lost. The essential nutrients would have spoiled, and humans would have lost one of their major sources of food. This food was not designed by chance.

Phytic acid is found in the bran of grains and beans. It combines with calcium and other minerals, and sees that our bodies receive the correct amount of calcium. If grains were balanced with much more bran than already present, we could develop calcium deficiency.[1] The correct balance is evidently extremely important.

What if by chance plants released hydrogen instead of oxygen, or animals released hydrogen sulfide instead of carbon dioxide? What if they released any of the thousands of other products produced by chemical reactions? The balance we find in "nature" would not support life. The design is very specific.

What if the tiny membranes in the endosperm by some chance had not developed? What if the biochemical pathways by chance had developed vitamin "2Q" or whatever, instead of vitamin E? If each of these unique circumstances were different, life would not exist.

David Green, of the Institute for Enzyme Research, University of Wisconsin-Madison, wrote:

> However, the macromolecule-to-cell transition is a jump of fantastic dimensions, which lies beyond the range of testable hypotheses. In this area all is conjecture. The available facts do not provide a basis for postulating that cells arose on this planet.[2]

Isn't random chance amazing? No! Random chance has no chance to produce the precise design we observe.

Did you notice that the "waste products" of both plant and animal life are fashioned into the plan or design? If animals didn't produce CO_2, plants wouldn't grow. The more animals there are, the more CO_2 is produced. Plants grow more rapidly and mature more quickly in higher concentrations of CO_2.

Plants produce oxygen. The more oxygen they have, the better animals grow. Could it be that this, too, was designed?

What a nice check-and-balance, hand-in-glove arrangement! Every member of the plant kingdom should be cheering for every animal that is

Spring flowers in Israel. Plants utilise the carbohydrates created by photosynthesis.

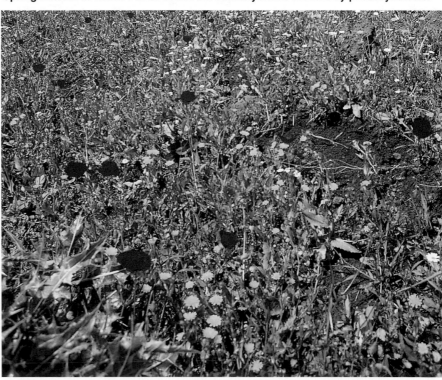

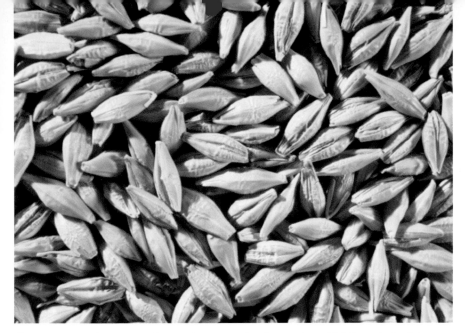

Corn—a general term meaning grains or seeds—is mentioned 94 times in Scripture.

born. Plants and animals need each other. Humans are not the scourge of the world—although they do need to be responsible.

Even if by humanistic definition science says God cannot be discovered by the rules science sets for itself, we have to admit that the complexity of grain is beginning to look like a design. And where there is a design, there has to be a designer.

Dr. Robert Jastrow, an evolutionist and astrologer, and director of the Goddard Institute for Space Research, wrote:

Most remarkable of all is the fact that in science, as in the Bible, the world begins with an act of creation. That view has not always been held by scientists. Only as a result of the most recent discoveries can we say with a fair degree of confidence that the world has not existed forever: that it began abruptly, without apparent cause, in a blinding event that defies scientific explanation . . . . All the details differ, but the essential elements are the same . . . . For the scientist who has lived by his faith in the power of reason, the story ends like a bad dream. He has scaled the mountain of ignorance. He is about to conquer the highest peak. As he pulls himself over the final rock he is greeted by a handful of theologians who have been sitting there for centuries.[3]

Word from the Designer

If God exists, and if He left an Instruction Book for us telling about Himself and His design, surely He included some information about food grains or seeds.

Corn: A Generic Term

Corn is mentioned 94 times in Scripture. "Corn" is a general term meaning grains or seeds—not the specific plant we know as corn. For example, neither rice nor oats are mentioned in the Bible; but the Hebrew and Greek words for "corn" can include many grains not specifically mentioned.

Wheat: The King of Grains

Wheat is mentioned 51 times in the Bible. Wheat is the *rex* (king) of grains. It was so highly valued in the ancient world that it was used as a measure of wealth. Today wheat is still the number one food or crop in the world. It has always been the chief crop in any country that has any tillable land.

Secular scientists found evidence that wheat was first cultivated in the Fertile Crescent, in what is now Iraq and Turkey. That makes sense biblically because Noah's ark landed nearby on Mount Ararat. Many scientists trace the origin of the various languages and nationalities to the same area.[4]

Long after this period, the Egyptians were sifting flour to make it whiter. The earliest histories of many other races also include references to wheat and baked breads.

Of course, we are more concerned here with the use of grains by the Israelites.

In Psalm 81:16, God promised, *You would be fed with the finest of wheat; with honey from the rock I would satisfy you.*

Wheat and other grains were offered as a reward for faithfulness.

The universal importance of wheat is probably earned by its *gluten*—the unique quality that allows dough made from wheat flour to hold together as it rises from yeast, forming a beautiful loaf. Gluten is found in the endosperm of a kernel of wheat. Although it is also found in some other grains, wheat has more gluten than other grains.

Barley: Tiny Grain, Great Gifts

When Jesus asked what food might be given to the hungry crowds who followed Him, Andrew said, "Here is a boy with five small barley loaves and two small fish" (John 6:9). Small gifts created by God and offered to Christ and His people can be used in great ways. Just as Jesus made this small fare feed a multitude, so God has made the tiny barley grain chock full of nutrients.

Barley can be used as flour for bread or crackers, as a sweetener and as a drink. In Britain, barley water has been used for centuries to help cure intestinal illnesses.

In recent years, much research has been done on barley. The nutrient content of young barley sprouts has been found to be loaded with minerals, vitamins and many other beneficial phytochemicals and antioxidants.

A Japanese pharmacist was the first to process barley into a powder used as a nutritional supplement. A huge industry has developed to sell this product. Minimal processing does not change the nutrient content, and the product is an ideal food supplement. (Beets, wheat, fruits, carrots and vegetable mixes are examples of other foods that can be processed into good nutrient supplements.) Many people take barley products and praise the pharmacist for developing it.

I have noticed a pattern in this regard. A person studies anything that was created for food. He or she shares its attributes with others, who are in turn helped. A reputation is gained. A business begins.

For example, *Green Leaves of Barley* is an excellent book about just this one entity in God's creation.[5] Many experts say barley is great for you. Others say not enough vitamins are contained in barley or its juice to be of much benefit. This may be true, but the total package of ingredients in barley has a synergistic effect because of its unique design. I believe it is a good supplement or food.

Other Bible Grains

Pulse is a grain the Bible mentions three times. The food Daniel and his friends ate for 10 days is identified as "pulse" in the King James Version (Dan. 1:12). In some references, pulse is identified as a sprout. Sprouts are nutritional gold mines of essential nutrients for humans and animals. They appear to have their highest nutrient content approximately two weeks after sprouting. Many healthy products are made by juicing the young sprouts and drying the juice at low temperatures.

Other definitions of the word translated "pulse" indicate that it refers to rye grain.

Millet is referred to only once in the King James Version. This is a nonfattening grain, a complete food, and has a good balance of amino acids. Millet is high in minerals, especially calcium; it is alkaline, and is easily digested; it can be eaten with or without the hull.

Millet grows up to 10 feet high in either rich or poor soil, and requires little moisture; it is therefore a valuable food crop around the world. In the United States millet is used primarily as bird or chicken feed, and the stalk is used for hay. The Hunza people of Pakistan once used millet extensively in breads, grits, pancakes and pilaf.

Rye is mentioned twice in Scripture. Rye and *fitches* are names for a kind of grain that also grows well where conditions are unfavorable for other crops. Rye has the greatest winter hardiness of all grains; it cross-pollinates easily; its nutritional content is similar to wheat. It also puts nitrogen back into soil, thus enriching it.

What a design!

Because grains are well suited for human consumption, many kinds of food are made from them: whole-grain breads, cereals, pasta and pastries; popped grain (as in popcorn); soups; juices and so on. These foods represent the very center of a healthful human diet.

Recent studies show that flax seed causes some breast cancers to shrink! It also lowers the incidence of breast cancer among women who are more susceptible (those who have breast cancer in the family and other factors).[6]

Raw Energy

Once when Jesus and His disciples were walking through the countryside,

He went through the corn fields; and his disciples plucked the ears of corn, and did eat, rubbing them in their hands (Luke 6:1, KJV).

The Greek word for "corn fields" is *sporimoi*. We would translate it "grainfields" today (as in the NIV).

Are raw grains good food? Sure!

They are alive with nutrients, fiber and many other unknown substances that are ready to make our cells thrive. Raw grains, nuts and seeds are probably the best way to obtain the beneficial oils designed for our cells. They are nutritional gold mines.

Jesus and the Breads of Life

Although raw grains are good for you, cooked grain products are also beneficial. Cooking does destroy some vitamin C and some enzymes, but it also breaks down those membranes we mentioned, freeing many vitamins and minerals and making them more easily absorbed in the digestive tract.

Jesus served grains both raw and cooked. He spoke of bread, giving it the highest respect, and using it to symbolize Himself as the source of life (see John 6:33-35).

Jesus also baked bread for His disciples. The disciples came in from their fishing and they saw Jesus having prepared,

a fire of coals there, and fish laid thereon, and bread (John 21:9, KJV).

(Eating foods when they are freshly cooked is the optimal way to benefit from their nutritional elements.)

Ripening grain. Raw grains are good food.

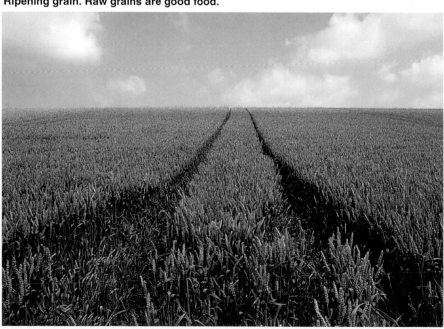

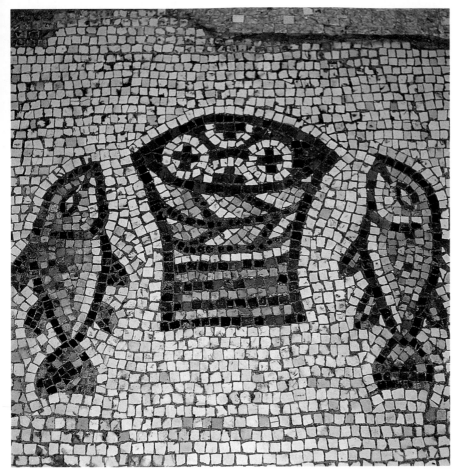

Mosaic of the loaves and fishes from Galilee. Jesus knew bread was a "staff of life".

Breads made from freshly ground grains can be particularly beneficial. The oils in grains are healthy; however, they do become rancid (spoil) through oxidation, often within 24 hours. The storage life of freshly baked bread is short unless it is stored at very cold temperatures.

The polyunsaturated oils in processed or cooked grains oxidize rapidly. That was probably why the manna God gave His people in the wilderness became rancid daily. Just as the Jews needed to gather the manna daily, so Jesus taught us to pray,

Give us this day our daily bread
(Matt. 6:11, KJV).

The idea is that we need to center our prayer for His provision daily.

Perhaps given a little more time the Jews could have learned to remove the oils and enzymes from the manna to produce white manna that had a longer storage life, thus removing the spiritual lesson—dependence upon Him—just as we have done.

Jesus knew that bread is a necessity for physical life, just as He is a necessity for spiritual life (see John 6:51-58).

Then he took the seven loaves and the fish, and when he had given thanks, he broke them and gave them to the disciples, and they in turn to the people. They all ate and were satisfied (Matt. 15:36).

Jesus' disciples knew the satisfaction bread can bring for sustenance and for fellowship:

They devoted themselves to the apostles' teaching and to the fellowship, to the breaking of bread and to prayer (Acts 2:42). *Every day they continued to meet together in the temple courts. They broke bread in their homes and ate together with glad and sincere hearts* (v. 46).

Today also, enjoying fellowship while breaking bread together is a highlight of an evening spent with friends or family.

A Symbol of Security and Love

In the Old Testament, some of Moses' last words were a blessing, and they included this prophecy:

So Israel will live in safety alone; Jacob's spring is secure in a land of grain and new wine, where the heavens drop dew (Deut. 33:28).

Think about it. The person who has a secure supply of pure water, grain and freshly squeezed juice has it made. It's not so complicated either.

Many years later, King David was on a battle campaign. Some of the people of the land knew that David and his army needed sustenance, so they

brought wheat and barley, flour and roasted grain, beans and lentils, honey and curds, sheep, and cheese from cows' milk for David and his people to eat. For they said, "The people have become hungry and tired and thirsty in the desert" (2 Sam. 17:28,29).

This probably represents an ideal list of gifts to bring when visiting family or friends, as well as a meal to offer visitors. (Contrast the poor visiting pastor today who is given cake, pie, ham, white rolls, bacon and shrimp—a feast of toxic or naked calories!)

"Which of you, if his son asks for bread, will give him a stone" Jesus asked (Matt. 7:9). It would be better to give our children stones than some of the foods we allow them to consume.

Speaking Loud About the Naked Truth

I once played in a state doubles tennis match. After the first set, I went with the other participants for water. One of my opponents asked me about my son, whom he had not seen in several years. I became enthusiastic in talking about my boy. We walked back on the court to start the second set. As my opponent started to serve, I took my position on the court. I had only one problem; I had left my racket by the water bucket.

Why does some loudmouth always bring the crowd to laughter at your expense? My problem wasn't really the loudmouths in the audience, but the fact that I had come to do a job without the equipment to compete.

The only situation I can think of that was more embarrassing was one winter when a friend stripped off his sweat pants while playing tennis indoors, displaying his new jockey strap rather than his new tennis shorts. That day *I* was the loudmouth, comforting my friend by saying, "This is the best showing you've made yet."

Nevertheless, I want to speak loud and clear about the naked truth of food that has been stripped of its designed ingredients. In particular, I want to show the effect of white flour, white oils and white sugar on our bodies. They enter the body assuming the task of keeping us healthy, but they are naked calories trying to do a job without the right tools and the right garb.

Stripping Away the Essentials

We have entered the match against poor nutrition by stripping away 90 percent of the natural nutrients and fiber found in grain. Because of our many health problems, the government requires that four nutrients be added back to white flour *after its natural nutrients have been processed out*. Then they call this flour "enriched"!

This is like sending a tennis player to the court without a racket, shoes or shorts, then giving him a headband and announcing to him, "Now you're prepared and enriched to win this game!" He would be embarrassed. If the grains God gave us could speak, they would be embarrassed, too.

No wonder the following chant is heard among the health conscious: "The whiter the bread, the sooner you're dead."

Another problem is that the iron used for enrichment cannot be ade-

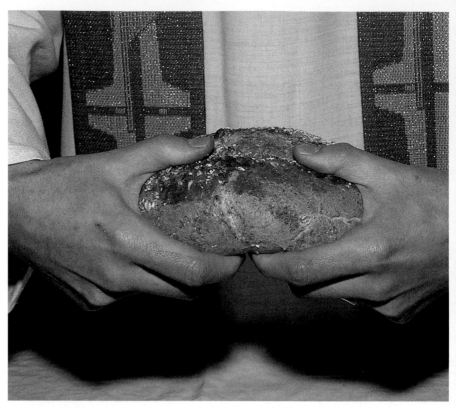

Jesus' disciples knew the satisfaction breaking bread can bring for fellowship.

quately absorbed in some forms, and in others it can be toxic.[7]

Sophisticated Enough to Be Ill

During the seventeenth century, rice polishing was perfected because someone decided it wasn't sophisticated to eat brown rice. The outer coating of the rice grain was removed to make it white.

Soon a disease of the heart and nervous system became widespread throughout Asia and other places where this fad became vogue. Christian Eijkman, a Dutch physician, noted in 1890 that the disease of beriberi was common among the wealthy who ate polished rice. He collected the wasted rice bran and gave it to beriberi patients, who promptly recovered.

Casimir Funk eventually isolated the vital ingredient in rice bran—thiamine. It was *vital* that this *amine* be ingested daily; and he coined the word *vitamin*.

Nuts, legumes, whole grains and leafy vegetables seem to be the best sources of thiamine. Meats also have thiamine. This vitamin is also used to enrich flour. The form that is best

absorbed, however, is not favored by the bread industry because it is water soluble. If I am being too subtle here, let me put it bluntly: *The nutrients being added to our food may not be useful, and may even be harmful.*

Why would anyone remove nutrients from perfectly good grains?

Of Lasting Value

Once I ordered some fresh whole-grain bread from halfway across the country. The baker taking my order warned that the storage life of her nutrient-rich bread wasn't very long. In my enthusiasm for this treasure (bread), I asked that she send it anyway.

It was summer. By the time the bread arrived, it certainly had enough nutrients to support life. Mold, fungi and plenty of growing things were doing well on what was left.

On the other hand, I've noticed that white bread can be left in our barn for days. The mice, birds and other critters won't touch it. A little whole-grain bread will have all kinds of life around, either eating it, eating the things that are eating it, or growing on it.

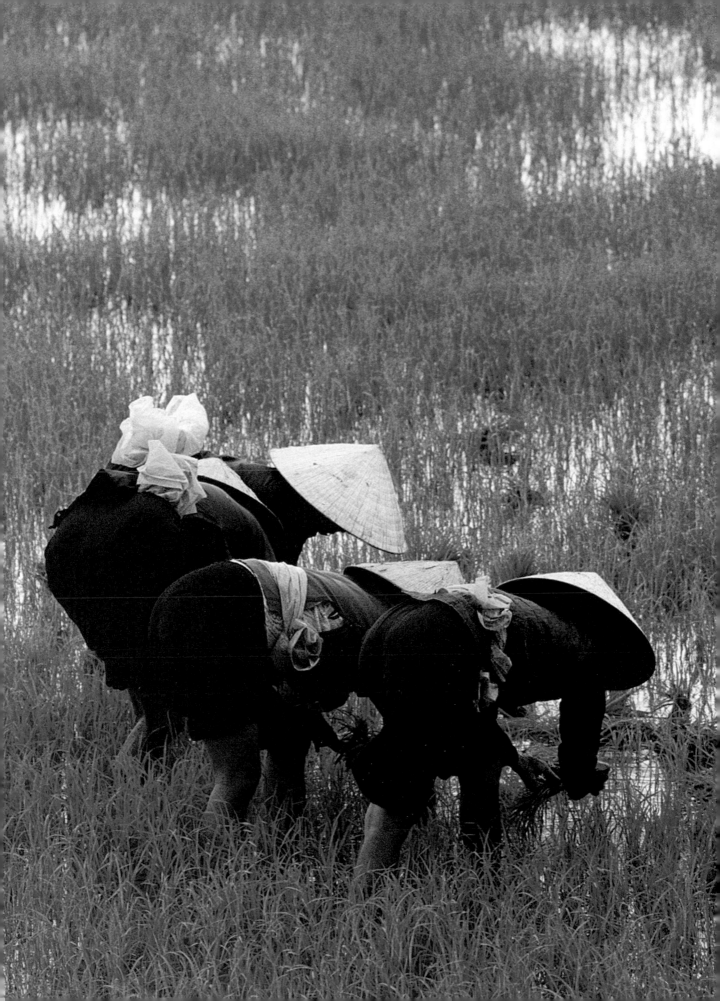

Fighting the Storage Problem

Granted that we want to be nourished by good bread, instead of having bread nourish mold and other growing things, consider some alternatives.

1. We can store the flour in the refrigerator, or eat the bread soon after baking. Good news: it remains healthful. Bad news: the cost of refrigeration.

2. We can kill all the bacteria in the flour or the bread with chemicals or radiation. Good news: more storage time. Bad news: the nutrients that support life are destroyed.

3. We can remove in the milling process all nutrients that spoil quickly. Good news: more storage time. Bad news: no nutrients, no health.

4. We can hurry up and eat the baked goods before the critters get to it.

The Milling Mess

Another way we have learned to make bread less healthful was discovered by the early Egyptians. They learned that sifting flour made the bread much lighter (because it had less fiber), and gave it a more delicate flavor. These lighter loaves were considered a delicacy, and they were the prerogative of the privileged.

Now, because of the sophisticated milling processes that have developed, white flour is available for everyone. All classes can enjoy its light taste—and cope with its resulting health problems.

What a bargain. White bread won't spoil easily, it looks prettier and it is lighter. Add sugar to the dough and it tastes like cake.

Many, however, say it is lethal. Should we require a warning label?

Twenty Steps to Poorer Health

Producing white flour requires up to 20 steps.[8]

The milling process is reported to raise the temperature so high that the grain is damaged by oxidation—another definition for burning. A good rule of thumb for checking a home mill or grinder is that the temperature of the flour should not be warm enough to be uncomfortable when you place some flour on your skin. Note what happens in a few steps of processing these wonderfully designed grains.

During World War I, shortages of grain in Denmark resulted in a ban against large bakeries milling grains. People had to grind their own whole-wheat flour. During these hard times, this one change dropped the death rate in Denmark by 34 percent each year the ban was in effect.[9]

Consumers seem to think that white flour is purer, and therefore more desirable. Many kinds of chemical bleaches have been used to meet this consumer demand—products that have the potential of being toxic to humans. One was taken off the market because it caused bizarre seizures.

Once this was discovered, the switch was made to chlorine dioxide. One of this chemical's by-products combines with uric acid to form a chemical called "alloxen," which is used in experimental animals to produce diabetes.

Other bleaches used to make white flour include acetone peroxide and benzoyl peroxide. These bleaches react with any remaining fatty acids to produce toxic peroxides and other harmful chemicals.

Unbleached flour is one step better than the standard bleached, enriched flour, but the best advice is to use an unbleached, chemical free, whole-grain flour. Unfortunately, just buying whole-grain bread at the grocery store won't do because if it is not refrigerated, it is missing the wheat germ. If flour has the germ layer remaining, it will turn rancid without refrigeration. *Some wise people buy a wheat grinder to preserve the nutrient-filled germ layer.* If you have one, share it with your friends.

A Principle III Warning

Principle III, you should remember by now, states that we should not let any chemical, food or drink become our god. Eating a variety of foods, and occasional fasting, can help prevent this problem. Grains must also be accompanied by a variety of other foods.

A teenage girl arrived at our hospital and was near death from anemia. She was not bleeding; but her bone marrow was not making any red blood cells. She was nutritionally deficient.

Was she starving? No. She was eating 2,500 calories a day. *But she was addicted to white corn flour.* What a disaster! Incidentally, all this despite the fact that the enriched flour she was eating had plenty of iron.

You would think the adage "Variety is the spice of life" originated in nutritional circles.

Despite the near perfection of grains, potential hazards exist if you rely exclusively on a single product. Some grains, legumes and vegetables often lack one or more of the essential amino acids.

A few years ago, some experts thought that vegetarians would display deficiency syndromes because complete proteins were not found in some grains, beans and nuts.

Grains and nuts may be deficient in the amino acid (AA) lysine, but have an abundance of the AA methionine. Legumes (as beans) may be low in the AA methionine, but guess what—beans are loaded with lysine.

Television news says, "Children are starving in Africa from another drought." The camera shows a small child having a bloated stomach, red hair, golden skin and swollen joints. He is dying.

The child, however, is not dying of starvation. He may be consuming 2,000 to 3,000 calories a day. He is dying of malnutrition. The tragedy is that his diet is limited to only one grain—corn or maize—which does not contain lysine. Some grains are sufficient if eaten alone, but others are not.

Dr. Cori Se Vais, who writes for *The Saturday Evening Post*, continues to send corn seed to Africa that produces a variety of corn containing lysine. This lysine-enhanced corn will stop severe health problems suffered in many parts of Africa. Legumes or other grains will also help.

Our needs will be met if we will eat a variety of grains, vegetables and legumes.

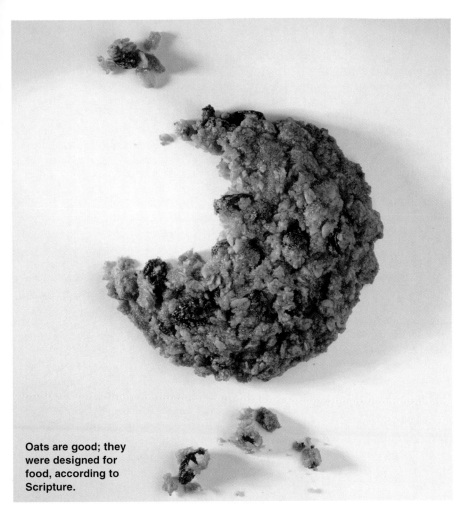

Oats are good; they were designed for food, according to Scripture.

God would not allow our health to be dependent on a single grain. If the power mongers corner the earth's oat supply, is anything else available to help those who have diabetes, heart disease and high cholesterol levels?

The wise, knowing that the Designer would not require us to devote ourselves exclusively to any one food, began to look for other good things created with fiber. Sure enough, beans, peas, buckwheat and other grains, as well as fruit, have been found to have plenty of valuable fiber, too.

How Much Fiber Is Enough?

When asked how much fiber we need, I often give the admittedly earthy answer that we need only to look into our toilets. As insoluble fiber passes through the bowel, it takes fat with it into the stool. Fat floats. So floating stools are a good sign that you have enough fiber. (You don't need to follow the example of my friend who left this message on my answering machine one day: "Eureka! I've had a floater!")

What About Oat Bran?

When the fiber craze was young a few years ago, oat bran was virtually worshiped with a religious fervor. Remember the story about the golfer who died and went to heaven? He went about marveling at the beauty of the golf courses there. Finally, in response to yet another outburst of wonder, St. Peter said curtly, "Well, you could have come 10 years sooner if you hadn't eaten so much oat bran."

The oat-bran craze was based on good information. The soluble fiber in oats reduced cholesterol and the incidence of heart attacks. Diabetics improved.

The sought-after ingredient was beta glucan, a polymer of glucose, which is indigestible. It passes through the intestine, taking with it fat and bile acids and reducing cholesterol formation in the liver.

People would buy anything containing the word "oats" on it. And if a product had both words, "oat bran," sales would soar. The price of oats and any product that contained oats began to skyrocket. Health nuts who joined this cult would buy products made of lard and sugar (candy bars) if the candy just had the word "oats" on the wrapper. I confess that I had a seat on this bran wagon, including the time I was studying my three principles.

Oats certainly are good; they were designed for food according to Scripture. Can a candy bar made with lard be made healthful by a little fiber from oats? Can sugar be good for a diabetic (or anyone else) simply because it is coating some oats? We should not neglect a balanced diet just to eat oats.

We are not to worship any created thing—including oat bran! Surely

The Legacy of Legumes

A chapter about legumes—beans and peas—would be similar to the preceding pages about grains. Only a few comments will be added about these wonderfully designed and complex foods.

Blessed by Beans

Legumes are edible seeds that are fashioned in a pod. They are a rich source of proteins and complex carbohydrates. They are low in fat, and the fats they do have are good for you.

Proteins comprise up to 22 percent of the calories found in legumes. They include most of the essential amino acids (AA), but are low in one AA—methionine—which is found in grains. The proteins include many enzymes made of thousands of sequenced, precisely crafted AAs that are all "left-handed." One of these proteins is a starch blocker. This enzyme will block the absorption of the abundant complex carbohydrates (calories) found in beans. If the person eating these beans needs additional calories, however, their pancreas and bowel release products that will digest the starch blocker, making available the needed amount of calories.

How convenient! Aren't we *lucky*? Or are we blessed? Only fools says in their hearts that there is no God (see Ps. 14:1). What a Design!

Legumes at Work

Legumes are also great sources of most vitamins and minerals, and fiber, but they do not have high concentrations of vitamin C or calcium. They retain most of the nutrients even after being cooked as long as 75 minutes.[10]

In many cultures, beans are mixed with grains. In Israel, two of the most popular foods are hummus (chickpeas) and tahini (sesame seed butter). On a trip to Israel I was served humus, tahini and hot sauce on pita bread. After I determined what this strange stuff was, I ate it like a newfound treasure. It was good, and good for me.

Soy beans are the largest legume crop in the world. The beans and their by-products are used for meat substitute, baby formula, flour, tofu, cooking oil, and on and on. The more this bean is studied, the more amazing it seems. Whole industries and great wealth have been built around raising and experimenting with soy beans.

What About Nuts?

Nuts are part of the same family as grains. The shell is the husk or chaff, and the "meat" is the embryo or germ tissue. Nuts are high in fat and in total caloric content; they have a poor reputation these days because of the fad that fat is always bad. Like the embryo of other seeds, the nut has a lot of the fat-soluble vitamins and essential fatty acids that repair damaged cells in the body. They are also a rich source of protein, although they may be low in lysine, as are some grains. Nuts have a low carbohydrate content, and only the chestnut has any vitamin C.

George Washington Carver took the peanut—a bean that is called a nut and is also a seed—and found 300 uses for it.

Getting It Right

Your health is worth the extra work and expense required to utilize the treasure of grains. It can be frustrating to read what humans have done to these wonderfully designed seeds; but after all, God warned us about that:

In the sweat of thy face shalt thou eat bread (Gen. 3:19, KJV).

Your health is worth checking labels to be sure products have nutritionally beneficial ingredients. Look for 100 percent whole-grain cereals, flours, breads, pasta, soups and pastries. Choose old-fashioned grain cereals.

It helps to be flexible and patient while searching for the food treasures God has waiting for you. When your spouse experiments, brag about him or her, even when what is presented is not the expected or the traditional. (Be careful—this can be carried too far. After a few bites of a somewhat peculiar offering one evening, I complimented my wife about this new delight. She smiled, and I thought I had pleased her—until she informed me that I had eaten part of the flower arrangement.)

Avoid any product labeled "enriched," "degerminated" or "denatured." All this means is that the product probably retains little of its original nutritional value.

Avoid products made with processed grains: cookies, cakes, pies, pastries, noodles, spaghetti and macaroni made with bleached flour or other processed items.

Also, choose cereals that are not presweetened. Many of them, especially those marketed at children, consist of almost totally "naked" calories. Some are 60 percent sugar, and most of the rest are made with white flour and artificial coloring.

The number of obese children in the United States has reached alarming proportions. Many are simply not getting an adequate variety in their diets. When nutrients are missing, our bodies send the signal, *I'm hungry! Get me more food!*

Obesity can be a spiritual problem as well as a health risk.

"Jeshurun grew fat and kicked; filled with food, he became heavy and sleek. He abandoned the God who made him and rejected the Rock his Savior" (Deut. 32:15).

Thank God for Grains

In short, grains, seeds and nuts contain many essential ingredients that will prevent illness, promote wellness and help recover health. By using them in accordance with their original design, and making only little changes in their composition, they will be of great benefit to your health.

After all, seeds were fashioned to bring forth life. They are a part of God's wise design; and we show our own wisdom when we recognize His handiwork in this area and add balanced portions of grain and seeds to our diets.

7. The Fat of the Land

Are those fats you've heard will kill you really that bad? Here are some answers that may surprise you.

It was 1944, and World War II was roaring. A young mother was wasting away with an infection diagnosed as tuberculosis. Antibiotics were unavailable. Her doctor prescribed (1) isolation, (2) bed rest, (3) exercise (eventually) and (4) *a diet high in fat.*

Surprising, but true! High-fat diets were often recommended by the medical profession during those years. Before you scoff, you might want to know that this lady recovered. She is my mother, and she has stayed on this diet through the years. Presently she is enjoying her great-grandchildren. Her actual description of the diet: lots of steak, eggs, breads, nuts, vegetables and (unfortunately) pork.

Fat: Killer or Healer?

In contrast, we are now told just the opposite—we must not eat fat because it is a killer. Who is right?

We are told we must not eat fat because it is a killer.

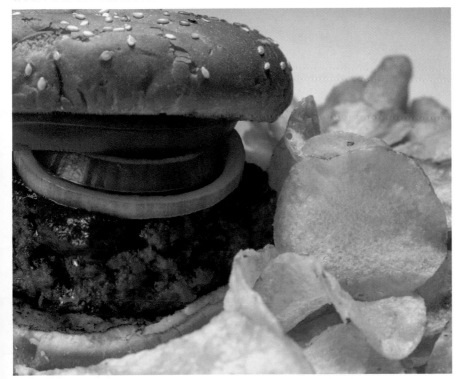

Could both approaches have some correct aspects? Before you accept the "fat is bad" fad, look at some additional information.

Looking at Lipids

Fats are "lipids."[1] The term "lipid," which is often used interchangeably with the word "fat," was created to include a group of compounds related (actually or potentially) to the *fatty acids.*

Lipids may be defined by what they have in common. They are (1) insoluble in water, (2) soluble in organic solvents such as ether and chloroform and (3) can be utilized by living organisms.

Lipids, therefore, include the ordinary fats and oils, waxes and related compounds. The principal foods contributing fat to the diet are butter, margarine, lard, vegetable oil, salad dressing, the visible fat of meat, the skin of chicken and the invisible fat found in cream, homogenized milk, milk products, egg yolk, meat, fish, nuts, olives, avocados and whole-grain cereals.

Whew! Quite a list of things to avoid, if we buy the "all fat is bad" fad. But read on.

Dr. Petr Skrabanek, in his book *The Death of Humane Medicine*, documents that the recommendations for a low-fat diet are based on spurious evidence.[2] He also believes that the "expert committee" findings that first endorsed anti-cholesterol, low-fat guidelines were based more on feeling than on fact. He quotes a group of experts, led by Jeremiah Stamler, exhorting that everyone of all ages should avoid butter, egg yolk, bacon, lard and suet.

In 1974, K. A. Oster said:
Recommendations of major dietary changes, with wasteful neglect of nutritious foods, such as butter, eggs, whole milk, cheeses, and beef, borders on irresponsibility and smacks of medical quackery.[3]

In spite of Oster's comment, the American Medical Association adopted this fad shortly thereafter. This action was taken with the best intentions for the health of the people of our country.

Choosing Our Lists Wisely

The list of classifications of bad foods began a frantic rush for other lists of good and bad foods. Too bad that those experts on the committees ignored the accurate list of good (clean) and bad (unclean) foods so carefully described by the Designer.

Of course, science based on the assumption that there is no supernatural could not use the Bible's more accurate list of good and bad foods. If you choose to believe that food is developed by a process of random chance, then man-made rules are as good as you can find. Following man-made rules for health, however, is so confusing that it is similar to one person standing on the stock exchange floor and trying to fill the orders of every bidder or seller at once.

Good food and bad food lists have become a fad. Committees that have high credentials are proposing a variety of such lists. It is easy to make their recommendations gospel–except for their contradictions! The problem is that although each of these lists contain some degree of truth, there are important contradictions from research and from other experts.

It should be said that the members of the committees making the many recommendations are motivated to help us! They meet, believe something has to be done and they make recommendations. As you know, however, on committees sometimes popular opinion rules, sometimes rank rules and sometimes truth rules.

From One Extreme to the Other

The 1930-1940s experts decreed that "fat is good" for you. During the past 50 years, various governmental agencies, medical societies and committees

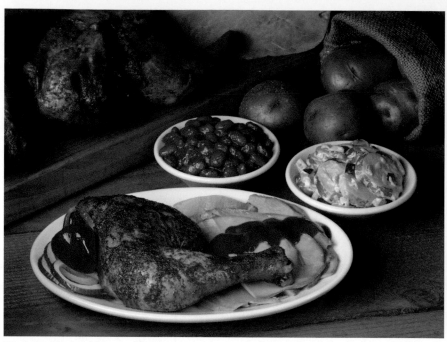

We have been told to avoid red meats, overlooking the fact that this is an artificial classification based on the color of the meat and not its content.

of experts have gone from "fat is good" to "fat is bad." Unfortunately, those of us who are interested in maintaining our health are totally confused.

Lord, help us! Show us the way.

A positive fact about all this: Our bodies need a wide variety of fats for hormones, cell membranes, transportation of nutrients through the blood and nerve conduction.

A negative fact about this fat advice: Toxic fats were allowed by the old-time diets. The cover fat of clean animals and all of the fat of the unclean animals are toxic fats.

The 1950s experts began to worry that dairy products were causing the increase in heart attacks and related diseases. Eventually they warned against whole milk, butter, cheeses and other dairy products.

A positive: Consumption of homogenized and other altered dairy fats decreased.

A negative: Butter, cheese, yogurt, kefir and other good foods were branded unhealthful. According to Dr. Mary Enig, a researcher from the Lipids Research Group of the University of Maryland, butter, coconut and palm oils have short-chain fatty acids that are used by the body for energy.[4] Because these fats are efficiently utilized, they are healthful unless they are overconsumed.

About Red Meats

The next attempt to curb health problems was the advice: *avoid red meats.* (It was overlooked that "red meats" is an artificial classification based on the color of the meat and not its content.)

Positive results: The meat of scavengers was included in the category of red meat, so bacon, ham, bear, raccoons, turtles, etc., would be avoided. Fried meat consumption decreased.

Negative results: Good food such as beef, mutton, deer, salmon and other flesh was excluded. Many essential amino acids and essential fatty acids are excluded unnecessarily.

The Cholesterol Conflict

Next on the battlefield's front line was cholesterol. This substance was considered bad because it was found in plaques that were blocking diseased arteries. Studies condemning cholesterol began to appear, but many other studies containing conflicting information were ignored.

The nation's cholesterol intake between 1900 and 1980 was basically unchanged. We would naturally expect the incidence of heart attacks to remain constant also. Yet *despite this constant intake of cholesterol, heart attacks have dramatically increased since the first one was reported early in this century.*

Many other studies question the validity of avoiding cholesterol intake. Only a low percentage of those who die of heart attacks have elevated cholesterol.[5]

A positive result: The toxic cover fat of animals was condemned. Most fried foods were looked at with suspicion.

A negative result: Eliminating cholesterol ignored the fact that it is important in the body's design. It is an essential component of many hormones, bile, vitamin D and cell membranes. It is also essential for the development of the brain. The myelin sheath of the nerves also depends on cholesterol. Both kinds of tissue are largely lipids, most of which is cholesterol.

Notice something else about cholesterol. Breast milk has six times more

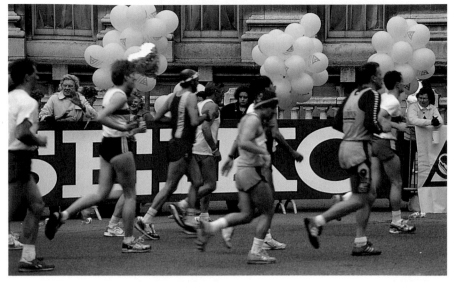

Only a low percentage of those who die of heart attacks have elevated cholesterol.

cholesterol than does cow's milk; soy milk has none; breast milk is best for babies. Even infants on low cholesterol formulas compensate by increasing the production of cholesterol in their livers. The level of cholesterol in their bodies remains low, compared to breast-fed babies, perhaps making them more susceptible to health problems.

The marbled fat in the flesh of clean animals can be a healthy fat.

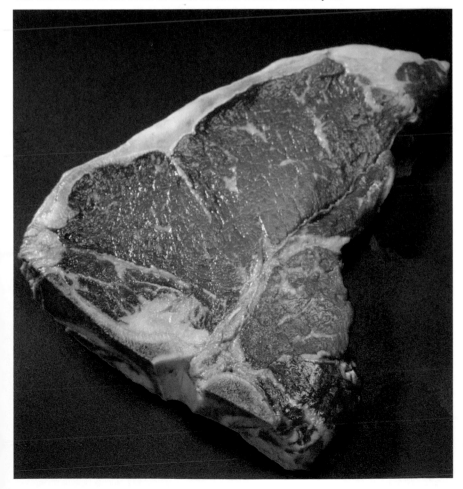

Aiming at Fatty Acids

The next target was saturated fatty acids. These substances are condemned for their presence in animal fats that were associated with cancer and hardening of the arteries.

A positive: The cover fat of animals—hard suet—is condemned in Scripture, so the modern advice to avoid this kind of fat is wise.

Negatives: (1) In the 1960-1980s, monosaturated fatty acids were also included in this category. Olives and their oil were considered bad. The rule also condemned many other foods such as butter, avocado, grains and nuts that contain the fatty acids designed for our health. (2) The marbled fat in the flesh of clean animals can also be a healthy fat. (3) The saturated fatty acids such as those found in butter, palm oil and coconut oil—those having short chains (explained in the following information)—were not differentiated from fatty acids having long chains.

Saturated buteric (butter) acid has only four carbons that are easily digested and utilized for energy. The body uses it much as it does complex carbohydrates. On the other hand, stearic acid has 18 carbons in its chain; it is stable and is used in cell membranes. Stearic acid causes health problems in the ratios of this fatty acid found in the fat that covers the muscle of animals, and also because it contains various chemicals, vermin or toxins.

About Polyunsaturates

Polyunsaturated fatty acids must be good, we suppose, because we have been told that saturated fatty acids are bad. Truth is twisted in this advice as well.

Positive: Foods containing high concentrations of unsaturated fatty acids such as vegetables, grains and nuts were recommended. This fad resulted in a sudden jump in the life span in the United States in the 1970s. This was good advice.

Negative: These fatty acids were processed from their designed grains. The polyunsaturates are unstable and easily become rancid when exposed to air, hydrogen, light and heat. Rancid oils are detrimental to our health.

Margarine was pushed on us because it had no cholesterol and was high in polyunsaturated oils.

Positive: None.

Negative: No evidence suggests that margarine prevents hardening of arteries. It is athrogenic (causing arterial disease) and carcinogenic (causing cancer). The hydrogenation of these vegetable oils saturates them and makes them solid. These oils actually become toxic when their structures are changed.

"Low" I Am with You Always

The most recent recommendation from the experts about fat is *low/no fat.* Contrary to their recommendations, however, a few good studies still fail to indicate an increase in longevity by reducing the total fat content in the diet.[6]

Positive: If this decree lowers the intake of rancid oils and toxic animal fat, it will help one's health.

Negative: If this decree lowers one's intake of the fats found in grains, nuts, oils and the flesh of clean animals, our health will be harmed.

At age 40, Nathan Pritikin had advanced hardening of the arteries. He drastically cut his fat intake to 7 percent of his total caloric intake, and

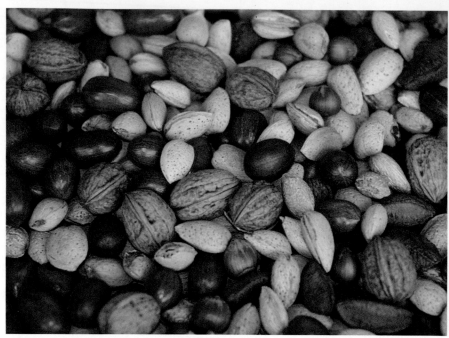

Foods containing high concentrations of unsaturated fatty acids, such as vegetables, grains and nuts, are recommended.

managed to drive his blood cholesterol level down to 95. Pritikin recommended the practice of eliminating as much fat as possible in his famous diet. Pritikin's low cholesterol count, however, did not prevent him from getting leukemia. Low blood cholesterol is associated with an increased incidence of leukemia and cardiac arrhythmia. At the time of his death, Pritikin had normal arteries, but eliminating essential fatty acids eventually was detrimental to his health.[7]

Jim Fixx, the runner, lowered his fat intake to approximately 10 percent, *and died of leukemia.* His actual death resulted from cardiac rhythm problems. Fats allow our hearts to beat safely. Fixx's blood cholesterol was 95. Low blood cholesterol is associated with an increased incidence of leukemia.

What I am saying here is eloquently expressed in an entire book, *Fats That Kill, Fats That Heal.*[8] The author, Udo Erasmus, is a Ph.D. researcher, professor and extensive writer about fat. Note how he expresses my argument:

The fact is that some fats are absolutely required for health, while others are detrimental. Some fats heal, and others kill. Whether a fat heals or kills depends on several factors. What kind of fat is it? How has it been treated—is it fresh, has it been exposed to light, oxygen, heat, hydrogen, water, acid, base, or metals like copper and iron? How old is it? How has it been used in food preparation? How much was eaten? What balance of different fats do we get?

If we get the right kinds of fats in the right amounts and balances, and prepare them using the right methods, they build our health and keep us healthy. The wrong kinds of fats, the wrong amounts or balances, or even the right kinds of fats wrongly prepared cause degenerative diseases that we call diseases of fatty degeneration. Other nutrients can also cause fatty degeneration, and so can lack of certain essential nutrients. We can reverse diseases of fatty degeneration by making appropriate changes in fat choices, preparation, and consumption, and by supporting these important changes with attention to other nutrients in our food supply.[9]

In contrast to the obvious wisdom of this statement, consider the "final" recommendations experts offer: *eat low-fat foods.* How much is low? Well, less than 30 percent fat. That is, 10 percent mono, 10 percent poly and 10 percent saturated fat.

How do you do that? No doubt, you're confused. I am, too.

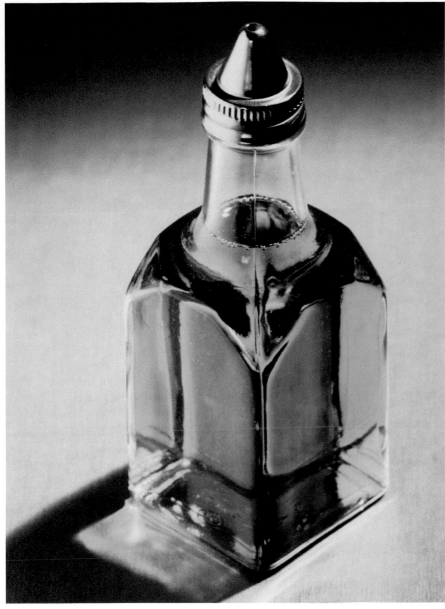

Studies have proved that olive oil is very healthful.

Warning: Experts at Work

Because any professional can be wrong, I urge you to let the Scriptures be your authority in this important area. In my own case, I will admit my fallibility by telling you something that happened to me when I was doing my residency at the Mayo Clinic in Rochester, Minnesota.

I was supposed to assist the chief of staff with some fluoroscopic examinations. A friend warned me beforehand that this guy was a tyrant. He would look for any excuse to chew out a resident, and was apparently on a mission to kick us out of the program. I replied that I had played football for a lot of years and was used to being chewed up one side and down the other by coaches, and that I could handle this doctor.

Admittedly, I was a little nervous on the morning we were supposed to do the exams, but I determined that nothing the doctor said would prevent me from doing the job so well that he would be pleased.

Well, the Chief came in and said, "Before we start, I want it understood that I don't want any conversation going on between you and the patient. I've written down everything I want you to say or do in the order I want it done. We have a lot of work to do. Let's get busy."

I said, "Yes, *sir*."

Well, the first patient came in, and I could not believe it. He was a guy from my own hometown in Altus, Oklahoma. He had been about three years behind me in school and I had sort of been his idol in athletics. He looked at me in surprise and said, "Well, Rex Russell! Look at you! You've made it to the Mayo Clinic. Isn't that something!"

Before I could say a thing, my superior stepped between us and put his nose right in my face and said, "You may have made it to the Mayo Clinic, but you're not going to be here long if we don't get the work done."

I don't know if you know what the "shimmering shakes" are, but as I replied "Yes, sir," they hit me. The fellow from my hometown could see I was in trouble, so he did not say anything else. I gave him a cup of barium and told him, "Stand with your back to the tall board (actually an upright table), and take three swallows." The exam began.

The next thing on my list was to instruct the next patient, a lady, to "go into the small cubicle, take all your clothes off and put this gown over your head, then come back and stand at the door to wait for your exam." I gave these instructions very firmly because I didn't want any more mess-ups.

Now, the Mayo Clinic never changes any of its policies; but they have now stopped putting gowns right by the pillow cases in the fluoroscopy rooms. Because, you guessed it, when the young woman came back in for her exam she had done exactly as I instructed. She stood there with a pillow case over her head—and nothing else.

At that moment my whole life passed before me. How was I going to explain to my parents and friends why I was kicked out of the Mayo Clinic? Would they think I was some kind of pervert?

My next words were, "Stand with your back to the tall board, take this cup in your left hand, and take three swallows." I was following my script very carefully, but of course the shimmering shakes were increasing in crescendo. I wasn't having much fun; but the lady dutifully drank from the cup.

After the exam, I ushered the young lady from the X-ray room back to her cubicle. I knew I was in for it, and was ready to bolt and run. To my surprise, however, the Chief said, exuding mercy, "Wait a minute, wait a minute. Russell, I've been here 25 years, and I've wanted to examine a lot of young women this way. But you've finally accomplished it. You're a keeper!"

Keeper or not, I had not given the right instructions. I represented an authority; I was sincere, I should have known what was best for the woman—but I pillow-cased her. She was embarrassed and I was embarrassed.

I tell this story to remind you that many experts are pillow-casing you with instructions about health. Some of my instructions may also be a pillow case for you. The only infallible guide to healthful living has come from the Creator, who alone knows what is best for His creation.

So let's ask what the Designer of fats has to say about the subject.

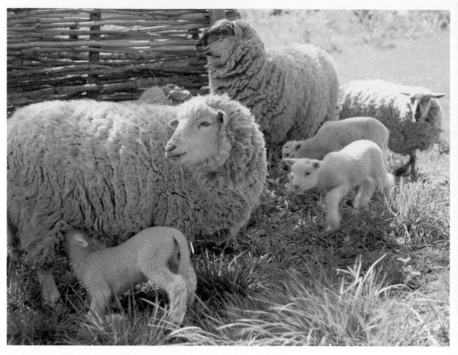

Among the "clean" animals are the ox, the sheep, the goat and the deer.

The Oil of the Olive

The word "fat" as it is used in these Scripture references is best translated liquid oils or "oil of the olive." Several years ago conventional wisdom said that olive oil, which is a monounsaturated oil as opposed to a polyunsaturated oil, was considered harmful to human health. Monounsaturated means the fatty acid has only one double bond.

Subsequent studies, however, have proved that olive oil is very healthful. It contains anticancer properties, leads to more efficient cardiac contractions and does not lead to vascular disease. Olive oil apparently promotes healing of atherosclerotic plaques. At Johns Hopkins University, studies have shown that olive oil is digested in a process similar to complex carbohydrates.[10]

So it was a sign of the Designer's love and care for His people when Moses told Israel,

For the Lord your God is bringing you into a good land—. . . a land with wheat and barley, vines and fig trees, pomegranates, OLIVE OIL and honey" (Deut. 8:7,8, author's emphasis).

Butter, Yogurt and Cheeses

Another fat God gave us to eat has earned the scorn of modern experts. He gave us

butter of kine [cows], and milk of sheep" (32:14, KJV).

Prophesy says the following about Immanuel, the son of the virgin:

He will eat curds and honey when he knows enough to reject the wrong and choose the right (Isa. 7:15).

Recent studies reported by Dr. Matthew Gillman of Harvard Medical School at the 1995 American Heart Association's annual meeting confirm that heart patients who ate margarine had twice as many heart attacks as those who ate butter. He was quick to emphasize that this doesn't mean butter was better, and

that the experts believed they needed to redesign the study.

I wonder why.

Before dismissing the word from the Designer about butter, consider the study of Dr. Beatrice Hunter, an enzymologist. She reported that when chickens were fed various kinds of fat, those that were fed butter had better bone formation and better insulin receptors than those that were fed vegetable oils.[11] Butter tastes better; it is better for your heart; and it is not implicated as a cancer irritator. Do we need more evidence?

Clean and Unclean Fats

Leviticus 3:17 says:

"This is a lasting ordinance for the generations to come, wherever you live: You must not eat any fat or any blood."

Why did God give this ordinance, if, as we have shown, some fats are good for us?

Again, Leviticus 7:23,24 forbids eating the fat of cattle, sheep and goats, and the fat of an animal found dead or torn by wild animals.

These passages must be taken in the context of clean and unclean meats, a crucial distinction made in Deuteronomy 14—in verse 3, Moses commanded:

Do not eat any detestable thing,

—and proceeds to outline the animals that are clean and unclean.

Among the clean animals are "the ox, the sheep, the goat, the deer, the gazelle, the roe deer, the wild goat, the ibex, the antelope and the mountain sheep" (Deut. 14:4,5; see chapter 8.) The internal, marbling fat of the flesh of these animals is healthful.

When Leviticus 3:17 forbids eating fat, it is not referring to the internal, marbling fat in the meat of clean animals, but to two other kinds of fat: the fat of unclean animals and the cover fat, including of clean animals.

I must admit that when I first read these bans against animal fat, which is high in stearic acid, I avoided all stearic acid. Much to my surprise, after many years of study, I found that stearic acid is also found naturally in many good foods such as olives, butter, grains and nuts.

It really doesn't matter whether stearic acid is present as long as it is used in proper ratios with other fatty acids found in the things created for food. Stearic acid is found in these proper ratios in beef, mutton, pork, butter, cocoa, coconut oil and peanut butter.

The ratios of stearic acid in the external or cover fat of beef, mutton, goats and pork—all forbidden fats— are such that the acid can cause the platelets in blood to become sticky, and to form clots. You would find this forbidden fat if you were to join a pathologist in examining the heart of a patient who has died of heart disease—the most common cause of death in the nation. It seems Psalm 119:70 has included these patients' lifestyles along with the proud:

Their heart is as fat as grease (KJV).

Stearic acid is related to oleic acid, the fatty acid found in olives. In the cell, enzymes can actually change stearic acid into oleic acid. Studies have shown that olive oil can reduce the risk of heart attacks by 6 percent within four weeks after starting its ingestion. Olive oil is up to 83 percent oleic acid and 13 percent saturated fatty acids.

If oleic acid is given in isolation, no significant health benefits are gained. Apparently the ratios of oleic acid with the other fatty acids found in olive oil provides the benefits of health.[12]

Fats and The Three Principles of Healthful Eating

Remember The Three Principles?

Principle I: Eat only substances God created for food.

Principle II: As much as possible, eat foods as they were created— before they are changed or converted into something humans think might be better.

Principle III: Avoid food addictions. Don't let any food or drink become your god.

Let's apply Principle I to fats.

Principle I: God's Created Design for Fats

Our cells use carbohydrates and fats for fuel. Both sugars and fats are like chains or trains of atoms having molecules attached to their sides. So fats and carbohydrates are structurally similar, although chemically they are different from each other.

At one end of these trains is a "caboose" called a "fatty acid." These substances are also used for fuel, as well as for transporting proteins—which are many times more complex than sugars or fats. Enzymes, which are necessary in helping the body utilize food, are one kind of protein.

To continue the analogy of a train, connectors called *bonds* link the "cars" of this complex train together. Fatty acids that have two or more of these links—"double bonds"—are called *polyunsaturated* ("poly" meaning "many"), and those having no double bonds are called *saturated* fatty acids.

God has built short-chain or double-bond fatty acids into fats such as olive oil, grains, butter and the internal marbling (not the cover fat or suet) of beef. By design, these foods are better for our consumption—because God designed us, too!

We have "fixed" the fats that God created to bring health and nourishment to our bodies, and in doing so have made many of them a health hazard.

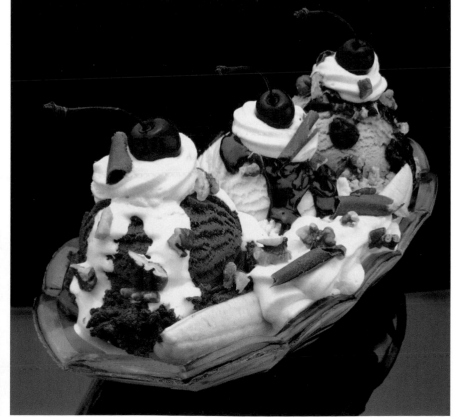

Principle II: Eating Fats as God Made Them

Proverbs 3:7,8 says:

Do not be wise in your own eyes; fear the Lord and shun evil. This will bring health to your body and nourishment to your bones.

Unfortunately, humans have not been content to eat "the fat of the land" as God created it to be eaten. Becoming wise in our own eyes, we have "fixed" the fats that God created to bring health and nourishment to our bodies, and in doing so have made many of them a health hazard.

Let us observe the process of making grain and nuts into clear cooking oils. This process employs chemicals, heat, air, light and hydrogen—all of which can cause denaturing, or rancidity in the fatty acids.

The process also tampers with the conformation of the "trains" described previously. Their shape is changed in ways that make it impossible for them to pull into the "train stations" God has designed in our cells. One of these changes is what makes vegetable oil become margarine.

Dr. C. Everett Koop reports about United States government studies that show nutrient deficiencies in as high as 80 percent of our population when only 12 of 45 essential nutrients were studied. *The study attributed 2 million deaths a year to nutrient deficiency.*[13]

Two Dutch researchers reported that 59 volunteers ate margarine, and as a result filled their blood vessels with fatty acids as harmful as the cover fat (suet) of animals. Other subjects, however, who ate only the fat of naturally occurring fatty acids found in olives, avocados and butter were not harmed.[14]

Unfortunately, an editorial in the same issue of the journal reporting the research advised that more research or labeling of margarine might be a good idea, and went on to warn against returning to butter.

The failure to eat fats as God created them results in the sabotage of the "warehouses" and "work stations" God has built into our bodies.

Think of these fatty acid "trains" as having from 4 to 32 cars trailing behind the engine. Each car is attached to the next by one or two connections (bonds). These trains run on extensive three-dimensional tracks throughout our cells. They pull in and out of many "warehouses" that have thousands of work stations ready with enzymes to modify their functions.

The modifications shorten or lengthen the fatty acids, or change the connection between the cars from one to two bonds or vice versa. These enzymes may break off a couple of cars for fuel (acetate) and burn them for energy to let the cell do other work. The cell may also add cars to a train to repair a cell membrane or improve some other function.

The cell can produce many kinds of trains, but they cannot produce essential fatty acids (FAs). These trains are important because many of the work stations are designed to receive only trains shaped exactly like these essential FA trains. These specifically designed work stations are perfect fits for the contour and shape of the trains. One change in a bond between two cars of the train will change the fit with the work station, resulting in a work stoppage or a strike until this deformed train can be removed. A lot of energy is required to remove a deformed train.

Refining our health away. Let's briefly survey what happens from a nutritional viewpoint when we refine the natural oils God placed in seeds and grain.[15]

We begin with a seed that is a rich source of essential minerals, essential vitamins, essential fatty acids, essential amino acids, fiber, lecithin, phytosterols and health-promoting minor ingredients. Even when we manufacture a fresh, unrefined oil—the highest quality of oil there is—all the protein and fiber present in the seed is lost, as well as some minerals and vitamins.

During processing, most of the remaining minerals and vitamins are removed. Lecithin, phytosterols and other components are also removed, and some essential fatty acids are destroyed. In addition, processing introduces toxic molecules resulting from the breakdown and alteration of fatty acid molecules.

Fully processed oils are the equivalent of refined (white) sugars, and can therefore be called "white" oils. Like white sugar, they are nutrient-deficient sources of calories, and also contain some toxins.

In making refined oils, the seeds are at first cleaned and cooked, perhaps for two hours at temperatures of up to 248 degrees. This destroys the seed covering and exposes the oils to air—starting the process of rancidity.

Next comes the process of expelling or pressing—subjecting the seeds to more heat and pressure. At these tem-

Dutch researchers reported that volunteers who ate margarine filled their blood vessels with fatty acids as harmful as the cover fat of animals.

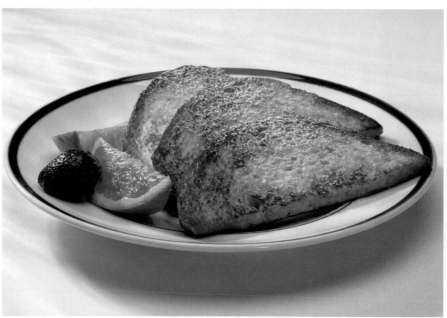

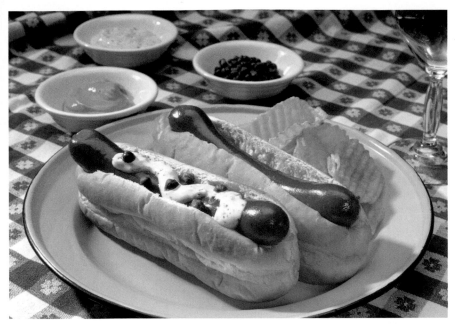

Nearly everything sold by the fast-food industry contains large amounts of fats.

peratures, it is estimated that rancidity progresses 100 times faster than at room temperature.

Then comes the process of solvent extraction, in which hexane or heptane (gasoline) is added to dissolve the oil out of the grain meal. The oil is heated to 302 degrees, evaporating most of the gasoline; but traces of solvents may remain, to a degree many health experts believe may affect us adversely.

Then, of course the oil is sold as "unrefined oil."

As if the extensive processing done so far is not enough, humans then degum, refine, bleach and deodorize the oil.

Degumming removes chlorophyll, phospholipids, copper, iron, calcium, magnesium and lecithin. Many of these products are recaptured and sold in vitamin supplements.

Some of this "refining" is done with a substance in a product you know by the trade name of "Drano"! Now is that a refined way to behave?

Despite all these efforts in violation of Principle II, however, some "impurities"—parts of the cell walls of the grain's endosperm—are still visible, causing a slightly yellow tinge to the oil. These remaining pigments include chlorophyll and beta-carotene.

So guess what. Next the oil is *bleached* with acid-activated clay filters at temperatures of 230 degrees. This causes toxic peroxides and conjugated fatty acids to form. The contour of the fatty acids is changed.

Deodorization takes place at temperatures of up to 518 degrees for 30 to 60 minutes. It removes free fatty acids and aromatic oils.

The result of all this? Clear, "white," odorless oils that are tasteless killers.

A blood test can establish the amount of harmful fat.

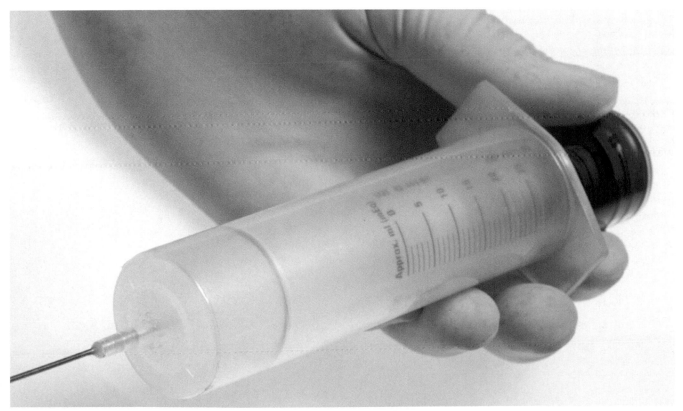

Principle III:
Avoid Addiction to Fats

Fat is one of the four foods to which people in our society are highly addicted. (The others, as you may recall from chapter 1, are sugar, caffeine and salt.)

Probably the best two things about the low-fat fad is that many rancid fats are avoided and addictions to fat are decreased.

The food industry, however, understands that humans love the taste of fats. That is why so many foods are deep fried. Nuts and potato chips contain hydrogenated fats. If you notice the products provided by the fast-food industry, nearly everything sold contains large amounts of fats (usually saturated, hydrogenated, fried, rancid, bleached, exposed to light and air), salt, sugar (naked carbohydrates) and caffeine.

Following our third principle, we can form another conclusion: Most of us have enough harmful fats in our bodies that they deserve occasional rests. Fasting is a good way to give them this needed break from damaging substances.

At times, the burning of fats and carbohydrates produces so many "sparks" and their fires, so many "chemical spills" and so much waste in our cells that for them to recover they need time to clean out the waste and repair damages. Fasting provides this needed rest.

Fats in a Nutshell

Healthful fats are plentiful, and are found in the unprocessed things God created for food. God promised His people,

"You can enjoy the fat of the land" (Gen. 45:18).

Enjoy . . .

Any fat found in a created food—nuts, seeds, fruits, vegetables and legumes—will be healthful. We can enjoy pure butter and unrefined liquid oils that have been protected from air, light, heat and chemicals. They have proven to be better for us than chemically extracted oils. The best oils for cooking are virgin olive oil and butter.

Even fat found in the marbled flesh of "clean" animals, birds or fish is healthful.

Avoid . . .

Nearly all liquid oils because they are severely damaged by the removal of nutrients and the addition of chemicals during processing.

If possible, avoid the meat of animals that have been overfed or given hormones or antibiotics. Also avoid their "cover fat" or suet. These fatty acids block the healthy functions of cells.

Avoid margarine and all solid vegetable shortenings because they contain artificially hydrogenated fats.

Above all, avoid the fat of all the scavengers.

Avoid high-temperature cooking such as deep frying. Cook by steaming or baking instead.

Remember that a healthful diet—including accepting the fats God has created for food, avoiding those that are harmful and giving our bodies occasional rests through fasting—are all ways of honoring the Creator. He loves you, and longs to have a personal relationship with you. Caring for your body—the temple of His Holy Spirit—is a way of showing your joyful acceptance of His indwelling.

As the psalmist sang in Psalm 119:92,93:

If your law had not been my delight, I would have perished in my affliction. I will never forget your precepts, for by them you have preserved my life.

8. The Meat to Eat

Did a loving God teach something about meats we should still need when He labeled some "clean" and some "unclean"?

I had been knocked flat on my back harder than I could ever remember. My muscle-bound opponent gloated over me as I picked myself up off the ground and strapped on my helmet again. I was playing for Oklahoma State University against the University of Colorado.

"Rex," my husky opponent said, "you'd better get ready, because you'll never know what's coming next from me." He was right. I could never have guessed what he was planning.

He stepped aside and allowed me to easily crash into the Colorado backfield, totally disrupting the play. The loud speaker announced, "Number 62 Russell makes the tackle for a two-yard loss."

My opponent said, "Rex, you did so good. Aren't you proud?"

Thinking he was paying me an honest compliment, I said, "Thank you."

The next two plays he crushed me. Then he would frequently let me go free again. What a bizarre game. It was off and on, hit and miss. I was confused. At halftime, my coach said, "Rex, you've had many great plays, but if you don't start playing a little more consistently I'm going to bench you."

I knew my opponent's coach must be yelling at him for his erratic play.

Meats Can Be Confusing, Too

I will save the part about how the game finished until the end of this chapter. Here I want to note that many Christians are just as confused about meats as I was about that game; and no wonder. We receive mixed messages.

"Beef raises cholesterol."

"Turkey is a good alternative."

"Chickens raised in crowded quarters are unhealthy."

"Fish is good for your brain."

"Shrimp can poison you."

If it is any consolation, the Early Church was confused, too. It was off and on. Some Christians considered meat to be good food created by God for us to eat, and others insisted that if it had been offered to idols it was as "unclean" as, say, the pork God had banned because of His loving concern for the health of His people.

The debate is reflected in Paul's letter to the Romans, chapter 14. Basically, Paul's conclusion is that eating meat or not eating meat is not a basic tenet of Christianity:

> He who eats meat, eats to the
> Lord, for he gives thanks to God;
> and he who abstains, does so to the
> Lord and gives thanks to God
> (Rom. 14:6).

Eating the *right kind* of meat, however, was not discussed. The argument in Romans 14 was about "clean" meats some Christians considered to be defiled because it had been offered to idols. The fact is, early Christians observed the biblical distinction between clean and unclean meats at least until A.D. 70.[1] The early Gentile Christian church observed the Old Testament law as well as much of the Jewish traditions until the Jews repeatedly rebelled against the Roman Empire during the last two centuries. Because the Gentile church was not in rebellion against the Romans, they separated themselves from the Jews by not following Jewish traditions and laws, hoping to avoid Roman retribution.

Why? What is so good about "clean" meats, and what is so bad about "unclean" meats?

Jewish people have distinguished between clean and unclean meat for centuries.

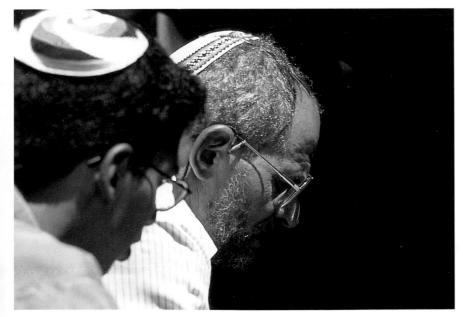

What Is Good About "Clean" Meats?

God said:

> "*You may eat any animal that has a split hoof completely divided and that chews the cud*" (Lev. 11:3).

He also said:

> "*Of all the creatures living in the water of the seas and the streams, you may eat any that have fins and scales*" (v. 9).

Birds other than scavengers were also pronounced clean (see vv. 13-20).

Why Health Is Inherent in "Clean" Flesh

The flesh of clean animals such as beef, and fish that have scales and fins, is ideal for the health of humans—just as we would expect from the hand of a loving Creator.

For one thing, meats contain proteins, iron, zinc and vitamins B6 and B12.

For another, clean animal flesh contains 3-omega fatty acids. These fatty acids are essential for life, and offer strong protection from vascular disease.[2] This is so important that we will spend more time on it later.

Many land animals God designed for food provide an additional benefit in that they generally eat grasses and grains that were also designed for food. The design of these animals' digestive tracts is especially significant in this respect. For example, a cow's stomach contains four rumination pouches in which various kinds of bacteria help to digest grasses and grains. These bacteria compete for nutrients, crowding out harmful bacteria, viruses and parasites. They also destroy many toxins before they reach the flesh of the cow.

The cow's digestive system presents its flesh with purified nutrients. This healthy rumination process allows deposits of healthy 3-omega fatty acids into a grazing animal's flesh. These fatty acids protect whoever consumes them from the harmful effects of triglycerides or cholesterol.

Great design!

Oiling the Body's Machinery

As we just explained in the previous chapter, some fats are essential to health. Various studies have shown that essential fatty acids such as 3-omegas fight arterial plaque and detrimental clotting in blood vessels. They also slow the spread of breast cancers, lower blood pressure and relieve inflamed joints in rheumatoid arthritic patients.[3] Fortunately, they are found in good supply in fish that have fins and scales, and in the flesh of cows, chickens and other clean animals.

These helpful fatty acids must be distinguished from the hard cover fat (suet) that is associated with arterial plaque. Dr. Floyd Byers of Texas A & M University has shown that longhorn cattle have 30 percent less muscle fat and 15 percent less saturated (very hard) animal fat than modern breeds of cattle; but they have a higher quantity of the 3-omega essential fatty acids.[4]

Additionally, cholesterol counts in longhorn beef are actually less than in the flounder fish—which is the ideal low standard for measuring cholesterol in animals. The longhorn may be unique, but other breeds that are kept lean probably could achieve the same numbers.[5]

Another example of design in the flesh of clean animals is the *prostaglandins* found in chicken,[6] and *alkylglycerols* found in clean fish. The flesh of other animals also have these compounds in lesser amounts.

In living cells, oils are changed into prostaglandins by specific enzymes. The prostaglandins in chicken have strong antiviral properties. (Maybe your mother's chicken soup *is* good for the flu and colds.)

Do you remember being frightened by the publicity about mercury being found in tuna fish? Actually, the alkylglycerols in the lipids of this clean fish pulls out the toxic mercury from its flesh. When we eat the fish, the alkylglycerols also remove mercury and other heavy toxic metals from our bodies.[7]

Alkylglycerols are unique in that they are oil-based, chelating agents—substances that grab and remove heavy toxic metals from our bodies. (They are also present in mother's milk and bone marrow.)

God's Provision of Protein

Probably the main nutritional value of meats is that they are great sources of complete proteins.

Our bodies have more than a million proteins that are specifically designed, shaped and positioned to do only one job. Many of the unique proteins have several hundred thousand amino acids coupled in a specific order known as their primary structure. The proteins also have a secondary structure that is helical (spiral), as well as a third structure—making it three dimensional.[8]

The complexity of these uniquely designed living proteins is truly mind boggling. Evolution by chance alone can't by any stretch of the imagination explain their origins. We who have finally abandoned that old theory are left with only a supernatural, awesome Creator—God. His word is good news for the health of all three dimensions of humans—body, soul and spirit.

Study on.

A Reminder of Principle II

I hope that by now, when you see "Principle II," you think, *Oh yes—we should eat the foods God has given us before the nutrients He placed in them have been processed away.* That important principle urges me to discuss a meat that has been widely proclaimed as a good substitute for beef.

What About Chicken?

Although the well-prepared flesh of the chicken as God created it is a healthful source of food (eaten in

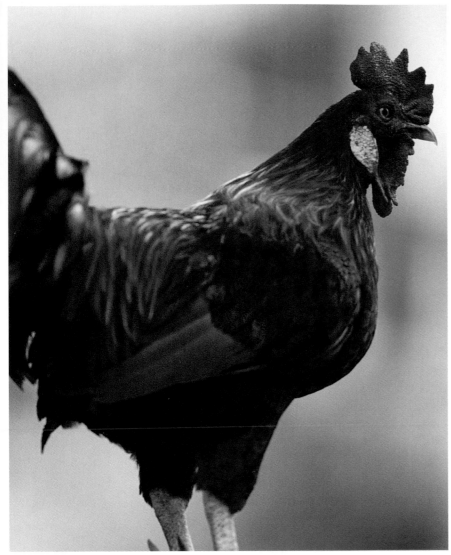

The well-prepared flesh of the chicken as God created it is a healthful source of food.

moderation), many tell me that chickens will eat anything. Their primary food, however, is grain and grasses. Their digestive system—the craw—is similar to the grass-digesting rumination pouches of the cow. Under normal circumstances, chicken flesh should be great. Under present food-preparation conditions, however, I see no advantage in eating them when compared to beef because most chickens are fed growth hormones, steroids and antibiotics.[9]

Unfortunately, the fact that consumers in the past seemed to like and want more fat in their meat prompted many in the meat industry to use such methods as selective breeding, over-feeding and chemical stimulation (hormones) to make animals grow bigger and faster.

Overfeeding results in excessively fat animals. If pen raised, an animal's fat content rises considerably. Wild turkeys contain 3 to 5 percent fat, versus 30 to 40 percent fat in domestic turkeys.[10] Pen-fed cattle contain 40 percent fat, versus 5 to 8 percent fat in grass-fed longhorn and some other breeds of cattle.

Dr. Byers at Texas A & M University also showed that the 3-omega fatty acids are changed into 6-omega fatty acids when cattle are fed excessive grain, antibiotics or hormones.[11] When the ratio of fatty acids changes, we lose the benefits of eating healthy flesh.

This offers a good lesson about Principle II and the importance of eating foods as God designed them. The healthful fatty acids are also changed when salmon are pond raised, when chickens are force fed and when eggs are laid by chickens who are fed commercial rations.[12]

Steroids and growth hormones given to animals may accelerate the maturity and increase the size of children who eat the meat. Earlier onset of menstruation in girls has been demonstrated when this kind of meat is introduced into a geographical area.

Antibiotics administered to animals for more rapid growth can increase the resistant bacteria humans are exposed to as well as the number of allergic reactions we may exhibit to drugs.[13]

Invariably, animals classified as clean have animal flesh that is good for us until we find a "better" way and mess it up, by adding hormones, antibiotics, pesticides and by over-feeding.[14]

Therefore, I recommend eating meat only from cattle that are raised without hormones, antibiotics or pesticides. This means we don't have to eat meat to survive; but if we do eat meat, it would be better if it were range-fed, organic, chemical-free meat.

Again: *Eat the things God created for food before they are changed.*

Precautions About Clean Animals

Although the flesh of clean animals is designed for our health, God did issue some precautions. Although cows (and oxen) were pronounced "clean" in the Designer's plan, we recall that their fat and blood were not to be eaten. Not only is the hard "cover fat" in many animals a repository for chemical toxins and parasites, but we have also learned of its danger as a plaque former in arteries and a cancer former in the colon and breast.

Also, eat only meat from animals that have been properly butchered. Basically, this means "treiberin"—trimming off the fat—and removing the blood from the meat. Butchers drain meat of blood at the time of the slaughter. Soaking the meat in salt water also removes additional blood products. "Kosher" standards include careful inspections of the carcass. All government inspections are patterned after the Kosher methods.

It is also important that meat be cooked properly. The meat Jesus ate was both lean—because eating its hard cover fat was prohibited—and broiled or baked. Cooking meat lowers the fat content, destroys some of the toxins stored in the fat and makes the meat easier to digest. Also, heat inactivates carcinogens—cancer-causing materials—in ground beef by releasing *anticarcinogens*.

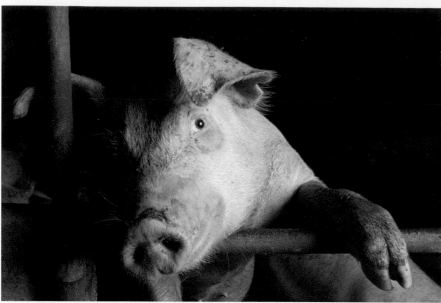

One reason for God's rule forbidding pork is that the digestive system of a pig is completely different from that of a cow.

On the Other Hand— "Unclean" Meats

The Lord said to Aaron the priest, *"You must distinguish between the holy and the common, between the unclean and the clean"* (Lev. 10:10).

The Hebrew word *chol* is translated "common" and means "shared by all"; or profane, unholy or defiled.

Although these terms carry with them the sense of ritual cleanness or uncleanness, holiness or unholiness, they also are connected with what is healthful or harmful to eat—in other words, with *physical* cleanness or uncleanness. So God wasn't just trying to curtail His people's diet for ritual reasons. Today as well, physical reasons remain for paying attention to what God said.

Our first principle says to eat what was intended for food and avoid everything else. The "everything else" is unclean.

Scientific Support for God's Wisdom

Much of the wisdom in the Divine Design for meats was confirmed by a 1953 study in which Dr. David Macht of Johns Hopkins University reported the toxic effects of animal flesh on a controlled growth culture.[15] A substance was classified as toxic if it slowed the culture's growth rate below 75 percent. In each case, the *blood* of all the animals Dr. Macht

tested showed up more toxic than the flesh.

The table opposite is based on Dr. Macht's study. His results show that *the lower the growth percentage of the culture, the more toxic the flesh.* Note that the flesh of animals and fish given to us by God for food are all nontoxic, but all forbidden animals lie in the toxic range. (Animals without percentage rankings in the chart were not studied, but are included here to provide a more comprehensive list of clean and unclean meats.)

Don't get confused! Any number above 75 percent is nontoxic, or clean.

This chart should make it easy for us to identify which meats we should choose to eat. It also makes it apparent we are eating many toxic substances that were not created for food.

The differences between clean and unclean animals appear to be related to their primary food source and to their digestive systems. Scavengers that eat anything and everything are unclean, not suitable for food, according to the Bible. Animals described as clean, and therefore good for food, primarily eat grasses and grains.

This examination of clean and unclean flesh could be a more revealing study considering today's modern toxicologic technology. A loving God protects His people by showing them just which foods are safe. He summa-

rized His will in Leviticus 11:43: *"Do not defile yourselves by any of these creatures. Do not make yourselves unclean by means of them or be made unclean by them."* Notice some of the mammals God made off-limits for human consumption:

"There are some [animals] that only chew the cud or only have a split hoof, but you must not eat them. The camel, though it chews the cud, does not have a split hoof; it is ceremonially unclean for you. The coney, though it chews the cud, does not have a split hoof; it is unclean for you. The rabbit, though it chews the cud, does not have a split hoof; it is unclean for you. And the pig, though it has a split hoof completely divided, does not chew the cud; it is unclean for you. You must not eat their meat or touch their carcasses; they are unclean for you" (vv. 4-8).

Note that an animal doesn't have to be a scavenger to be unclean. Horses and rabbits, for example, are unclean because they do not have split hooves. Although they are considered to be good food in some countries, studies have shown that horse meat often contains viruses and parasites.[16] Rabbits, as innocent as they appear, are the cause of tularemia (an infectious disease) in humans.

Quadrupeds (Four Footed)

CLEAN		UNCLEAN	
(Cloven-hoofed and cud chewing)		black bear	59%
calf	82%	camel	41%
deer	98%	cat	62%
goat	90%	coney (guinea pig)	46%
ox	91%	dog	62%
sheep	94%	fox (silver)	58%
		grizzly bear	55%
		ground hog	53%
		hamster	46%
		horse	39%
		opossum	53%
		rabbit	49%
		rat	55%
		rhinoceros	60%
		squirrel	43%
		swine	54%

Fish

CLEAN		UNCLEAN	
(With scales and fins)		(Without scales and fins)	
black bass	80%	catfish	48%
black drum	105%	clams	
bluefish	80%	crabs	
carp	90%	eel	40%
channel bass	80%	lobster	
chub	91%	octopus	
cod	98%	oysters	
croaker	90%	porcupine fish	60%
flounder	83%	puffer	51%
flying fish	87%	sand skate	59%
goldfish	88%	scallops	
haddock	80%	shark (dogfish)	62%
hake	98%	shrimp	
halibut	82%	squid	
herring	100%	stingray	46%
kingfish	83%	toad fish	49%
mullet	87%		
pike	98%		
pompano	110%		
porgy	80%		
rainbow trout	81%		
rock bass	100%		
salmon	81%		
smelt	90%		
sea bass	103%		
shad	100%		
Spanish mackerel	98%		
spot	80%		
sturgeon	87%		
tuna (bluefin)	88%		
white perch	81%		
Carolina whiting	84%		
yellow perch	87%		

Birds

CLEAN		UNCLEAN	
goose	85%	bat	
chicken	83%	cormorant	
coot	88%	crow	46%
duck	98%	eagle	
pigeon	93%	falcon	
quail	89%	hawk	
swan	87%	heron	
turkey	85%	ibis	
		kite	
		nighthawk	
		osprey	
		ostrich	
		owl	62%
		pelican	
		raven	
		red-tail hawk	36%
		sparrow hawk	63%
		sea gull	
		stork	
		vulture	

Insects

CLEAN		UNCLEAN
(Winged, hopping, with four legs)		(All others)
cricket		
grasshopper		
locust		

The Perils of Pork

Jesus, as one who was "born under [the] law" (Gal. 4:4), did not eat pork. One time He used pigs as a dumping ground for demons, evicting the demons and destroying the swine (see Matt. 8:28-32). This event occurred after weeks of healing various diseases.

One reason for God's rule forbidding pork is that the digestive system of a pig is completely different from that of a cow. It is similar to ours, in that the stomach is very acidic. Pigs are gluttonous, never knowing when to stop eating. Their stomach acids become diluted because of the volume of food, allowing all kinds of vermin to pass through this protective barrier. Parasites, bacteria, viruses and toxins can pass into the pig's flesh because of overeating. These toxins and infectious agents can be passed on to humans when they eat a pig's flesh.

Were there any benefits? In the *Biblical Archeological Review*, Jane Cahill examined the toilets of a Jewish household in Jerusalem, finding no parasites nor infectious agents, but only pollen from the many fruits, vegetables and herbs they had eaten. A similar study about Egyptians revealed eggs from Schistosoma, Trichinella, wire worm and tapeworms, all found in pork. All of these organisms cause significant chronic diseases.[17]

In what is probably a strong illustration of the perils of pork, at one time no cases of trichinosis had been reported in the country of Bolivia for several years.[18] However, 25 percent of pigs tested were infested with trichinosis. People working on these farms and the population eating the pigs were also found to be positive for infestation with this parasite. The primary symptoms of this infection include muscle pain, headaches, fever and swelling in the extremities.[19] These are all nonspecific symptoms that do not necessarily indicate any one disease. Although this may explain why the trichinosis had not been diagnosed in Bolivia for several years, it is strong circumstantial evidence that many people became ill because of pork.

Is it unfair to pose this question? Have you ever had either unexplained muscle pain, headache, fever or swelling?

Dr. W. J. Zimmerman reviewed the diaphragm muscle from multiple autopsies done in the United States in the late 1960s, and reported that trichinosis was not an unusual finding.[20] It is well accepted that illnesses caused by parasites have a significant economic effect worldwide.

In the United States, three of the six most common food-borne parasitic diseases of humans are associated with pork consumption. These include toxoplasmosis, taeniasis or cysticercosis (caused by the pork tapeworm Taenia solium) and trichinellosis.

In Japan, the source of these infections was traced to the flesh of pigs, bears,[21] horses, raccoons and foxes.[22] All of these animals are listed in Scripture as putrid or unclean.

Swine are also good incubators of toxic parasites and viruses—although the animal doesn't usually appear to be ill while carrying these diseases. A scientist at the University of Giessen's Institute for Virology in Germany

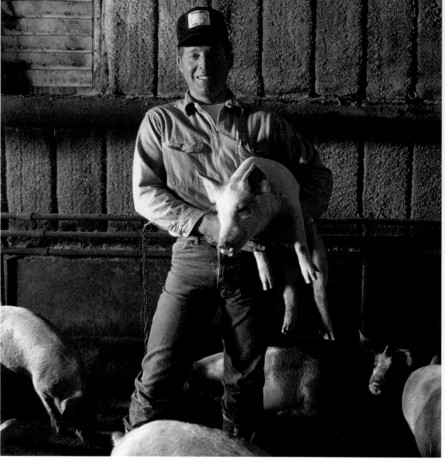

Just handling swine has an element of risk.

showed in a study of worldwide influenza epidemics that pigs are the one animal that can serve as a mixing vessel for new influenza viruses that may seriously threaten world health.

If a pig is exposed to a human's DNA virus and then a bird's virus, the pig mixes the two viruses—developing a new DNA virus that is often extremely lethal for humans. These viruses have already caused worldwide epidemics and destruction. Virologists have concluded that if we do not find a way to separate humans from pigs, the whole earth's population may be at risk.[23]

The 1942 Yearbook of Agriculture reported that 50 diseases were found in pigs, and many of these diseases were passed on to humans by eating the pig's flesh.[24]

Additionally, just handling swine has an element of risk. A large hog-raising facility in the area where I live wisely requires its employees to wear gloves, masks and protective clothing while working in the pig barns. The workers are required to shower each day before going home.

Little wonder that God would

inspire His prophet to include eating pork among the disobedient acts of stubborn people who in addition to idolatry and conjuring spirits of the dead,

"continually provoke me to my very face,...who eat the flesh of pigs, and whose pots hold broth of unclean meat" (Isa. 65:3,4).

Unclean Water Life

Because the Israelites lived near the Mediterranean Sea and around other bodies of water, God instructed them regarding many forms of sea life:

"Of all the creatures living in the water of the seas and the streams, you may eat any that have fins and scales. But all creatures in the seas or streams that do not have fins and scales—whether among all the swarming things or among all the other living creatures in the water—you are to detest" (Lev. 11:9,10).

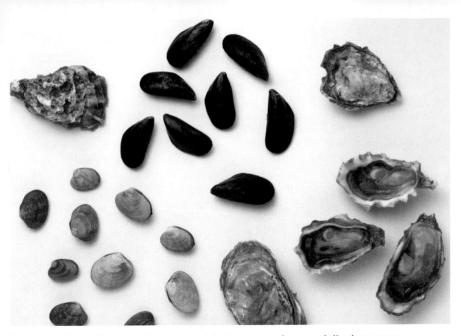

The meat of shellfish—shrimp, crabs, lobsters, etc.—is especially dangerous.

Although Jesus was "the end of the law for righteousness" (see Rom. 10:4), He recognized and called attention to the need to distinguish between good and bad fish. He spoke about unclean fish in a parable of the kingdom of God in Matthew 13:

"Once again, the kingdom of heaven is like a net that was let down into the lake and caught all kinds of fish. When it was full, the fishermen pulled it up on the shore. Then they sat down and collected the good fish in baskets, but threw the bad away" (vv. 47,48).

The Dangers of Shellfish

It has long been recognized that the meat of shellfish—shrimp, crabs, lobsters, etc.—is especially dangerous. Many illnesses, including instant paralysis, devastate some people every day as a result of eating shellfish.[25]

The largest cholera outbreak in the United States occurred in Louisiana from August through October 1986. (The symptoms of cholera are explosive diarrhea, leading to rapid dehydration, unconsciousness, hypotension and death.) What did the stricken people eat? The incriminating meals were found to include rice noodles with shrimp, pork, vegetables, mussel soup, pig blood coagulated with vinegar, and salty brine shrimp with mixed vegetables.

Shellfish can be placed in a body of water that is contaminated with cholera bacteria, and they will purify the water. Shrimp, oysters, crab, scallops and mussels are particularly efficient at this. They filter large volumes of water every day. Sewage laden with chemicals, toxins and harmful bacteria, parasites and viruses become concentrated in those shellfish.

The cause of cholera outbreaks in several areas has been traced to contaminated shrimp, crab, oysters and clams. A recent outbreak of cholera in Central America was related to shellfish ingestion. All this led one researcher to say, "By far the single greatest danger posed by seafood is from raw shellfish."[26] The flesh of shellfish is where the disease-causing organisms are found.

Although crabs are the most important vehicle for one strand of cholera infection in the United States, shrimp and oysters from the Gulf Coast are also vehicles of transmission for these diseases.

A case-control study has shown that stricken patients were more likely than neighborhood-control subjects without disease to have eaten cooked crabs or cooked or raw shrimp during the week before the illness.

These findings occur worldwide. In another study, 20 percent of 559 volunteers who were not sick, but who regularly ate shellfish, had serological (changes in the blood indicating exposure to cholera bacteria) evidence of cholera.[27] They had apparently been infected by the foods they ate. The volunteers' natural resistance, or possibly a less toxic strain of cholera bacteria, probably prevented severe symptoms or death.

Reading all this, you might not be surprised to learn that the state Legislature of California proposed a law requiring the food industry to label shellfish with a message warning: "This food may be dangerous to your health." Why? In a single year, 50 deaths and many hospitalizations were found to have been caused by eating shellfish.[28]

"Defiling" ourselves by eating shellfish—or any other unclean flesh—is as much a game of Russian roulette as is sexual misconduct.

Relax. You are learning the way to avoid such problems.

Animals That Crawl in the Dirt

Other animals that were off-limits are listed in Leviticus 11:

"Of the animals that move about on the ground, these are unclean for you: the weasel, the rat, any kind of great lizard, the gecko, the monitor lizard, the wall lizard, the skink and the chameleon" (vv. 29,30).

A few years ago, a sudden population explosion of armadillos—the cute little anteater all covered with scales—occurred in Texas and other southern states. Someone recommended that the armadillo be used for food. Special recipes were designed to make them tasty. Food engineers, trained to find new supplies from which to feed the world's hungry, seriously considered the armadillo.

If you were on a budget and could get this meat cheaply, would you go for it? You would be wise to first evaluate it with The Three Principles.

Armadillos do not pass Principle I. They are not a food God created for humans. They are not to be eaten, because they do not have split hooves nor do they chew the cud. You don't even have to look at the other principles. What have you missed by being obedient to the Bible? Several people in East Texas were infected with type M leprosy after enjoying themselves at armadillo feasts.[29]

Recommendations: Eat only "clean" flesh. Eat organic or chemically free animal flesh. Enjoy.

The Threat of Viruses

Other unclean animals can possibly change benign viruses into toxic viruses. Often when a virus moves from one species in which it is harmless to another species, the new species can be devastated by the new variant of virus. The green monkey—another unclean animal—has been shown to do this in connection with the HIV virus.[30] (The swine flu epidemics from Hong Kong that now have occurred worldwide have been documented to develop by this mechanism.)

I hate to be an alarmist, but genetic engineering may be producing new toxic strains in our labs rather than just in the unclean animals. Some believe the Gulf War syndrome, a wasting disease affecting the immune system, is caused by a laboratory combination of a virus and bacteria.[31]

Viruses carried by unclean animals apparently contribute silently to many other health problems. Dr. David Hajjar found that the herpes virus causes ulcers in our arteries, leading to atherosclerosis. Other viruses have been found to cause rheumatoid arthritis and juvenile diabetes.[32]

Infectious diseases and strange, uncontrollable epidemics are occurring all over the world, spawning novels and movies—and their plots aren't fanciful. Something like one-third of the world's population is said to be at risk.

So many people today violate these guidelines that the question is not "Why do we get sick?" but "Why aren't we all sick most of the time?"

Doesn't Cooking Make It Safe?

Some people tell me that unlike people in Bible times, we cook meat much better today, and that this renders even unclean meats harmless. One Bible commentary claimed that pork was forbidden in the Old Testament because it was eaten without being cooked, thus passing trichinosis to humans. The author thought that because we now cook meat, we no longer need to follow that law.

In my opinion this statement is incorrect. Sophisticated ovens and cooking devices have been found in the most ancient archeological ruins, including most of the Israelites' ruins.

They understood that cooking meat is certainly important. Can we safely assume that diseases caused by unclean animals have disappeared because we now cook things better?

Who can bring a clean thing out of an unclean? not one
(Job 14:4, KJV).

Even the microwave oven heats meat unevenly, allowing bacteria and parasites (such as trichinosis) to survive in meat. Many outbreaks of vicious infections have developed in so-called cooked food. If the food is unclean, don't count on cooking it to protect you. Some of the most toxic poisons are not destroyed by heat.[33]

A sobering report from Scotland revealed that food poisoning by toxins, virus or bacteria occurred in spite of thorough inspection at every stage of food preparation, including handling and cooking.[34]

Food poisoning by toxins, virus or bacteria can occur in spite of thorough inspection at every stage of food preparation, including handling and cooking.

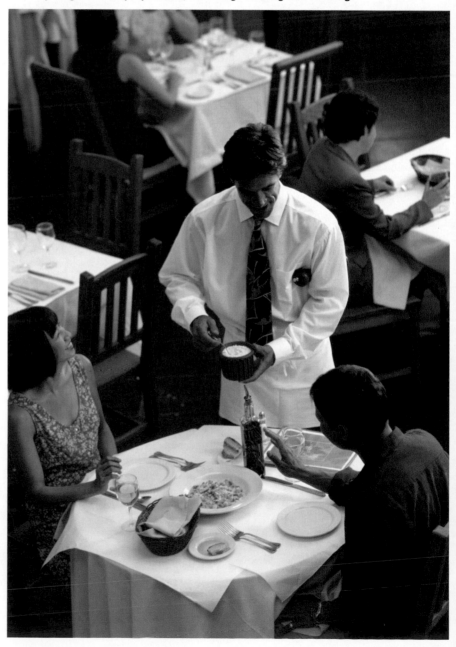

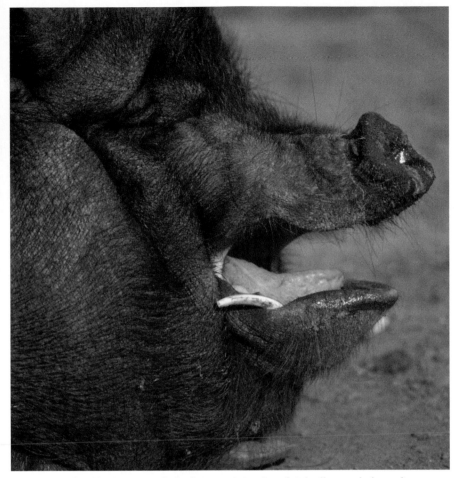

Pigs are unhealthy because their diet consists of society's disease-laden refuse.

earth, and shellfish and catfish are ideally designed to purify water, we don't want to eat what they clean up! But aren't we?

You may be surprised to find that giving up scavengers will be easier than you think!

Principle III: Too Much Meat?

Eating too much meat—both unclean meat or supercharged, chemical-enhanced, overprocessed clean meat—can cause illness. Even perfectly designed, clean, unprocessed meat can be easily overdone. We just do not need the huge amounts of protein most of us consume. Many symptoms can usually be cleared up by the partial fast (see chapter 5), by giving up unclean meat all together and clean meat for most meals.

Otherwise healthy and well-nourished patients who had rheumatoid arthritis showed significant clinical improvement after fasting for 7 to 10 days.[36] The improvement is reversible, so these patients lost ground when they started eating again. The authors of the study were at a loss to explain their findings. A good place to start is the information about clean and unclean meats given by the Designer of those swollen joints and of that toxic meat.

If arthritis is caused by toxic flesh or processed meats, a vegetarian diet should relieve the arthritis for a prolonged period. Please read part of an abstract from a scientific article about the subject:

Fasting is an effective treatment for rheumatoid arthritis, but most patients relapse on reintroduction of food. The effect of fasting followed by one year of a vegetarian diet was assessed in a randomised, single-blind controlled trial. The benefits in the diet group were still present after one year, and evaluation of the whole course showed significant advantages for the diet group in all measured indices. This dietary regimen seems to be a useful supplement to conventional medical treatment of rheumatoid

Why Were Scavengers Designed?

Why were scavengers created if not to eat? For one thing, they serve a useful role just cleaning up the place.

Many unclean animals, however, notably pigs and shellfish, are unhealthy because their diet consists of society's disease-laden refuse.

As is well known, pigs will eat anything and everything. They were designed to clean up decaying flesh and pollution. Pigs have eaten Philadelphia's garbage and sewage for more than 100 years, saving the city $3 million a year in landfill costs. This is a wise use of hogs. They are designed to clean our environment.

Even when stacked in cages, piglets thrive on offal when only the pig in the top cage receives food. Farmers have increased their profits by feeding free raw sewage to pigs. Chicken farmers often keep a hog so they can dispose of dead chickens without having to bury them.

Among commonly eaten fish, catfish—unclean because they do not have scales—always show the highest levels of contamination in chemically polluted water. After chemical spills, local fishermen are warned not to eat catfish.

A local peach farmer sprayed his crop; then an immediate rain followed. The rainwater containing the recently applied insecticide ran into his pond. The catfish did their job, cleaning the water by sucking up the pesticide; but because of their efficiency, most of them floated to the top of the pond dead. None of the fish that had fins and scales died.

Consumer Reports tested fish bought in multiple markets in the United States. Fish are considered spoiled when bacteria counts are greater than 10 million per gram of flesh. Nearly all catfish had counts that went off the scale at 27 million per gram, even when properly prepared.[35]

So although swine help clean the

arthritis.[37]

Most people in the United States would benefit from decreased consumption of meats, fasting from it for a few days or eating it only for celebrations.

What About Eggs?

Eggs are similar to meat in that they are also a rich source of protein. As everyone knows, however, they have received a great deal of bad press in the various reports of the dangers of cholesterol.[38]

The Bible provides little information about eggs as a food. One reference appears in the book of Job:

"Is tasteless food eaten without salt, or is there flavor in the white of an egg? I refuse to touch it; such food makes me ill"
(Job 6:6,7).

It isn't clear whether Job refused to eat all egg whites, or only unsalted egg whites or whether he ate only egg whites without eating the yoke.

In the New Testament, Jesus referred to eggs as a "good gift":

"Which of you fathers, if your son asks for a fish, will give him a snake instead? Or if he asks for an egg, will give him a scorpion? If you then, though you are evil, know how to give good gifts to your children, how much more will your Father in heaven give the Holy Spirit to those who ask him!" (Luke 11:11-13).

I am sure Jesus was referring here to hen eggs. I would not recommend dinosaur eggs or other unclean eggs.

Studies do indicate that the yoke of the egg has a considerable amount of cholesterol, but the yolk also contains lecithin, which breaks down cholesterol and probably negates any ill effects.

Challenge studies done at the University of Missouri showed some good effects from eating eggs.[39] Three eggs a day were ingested by 70 people during a three-month period. Their blood tests showed an elevation of high density cholesterol—"good cholesterol"—while eating eggs. Their triglyceride levels were unchanged.

At the American Heart Association meeting in Anaheim, California, in

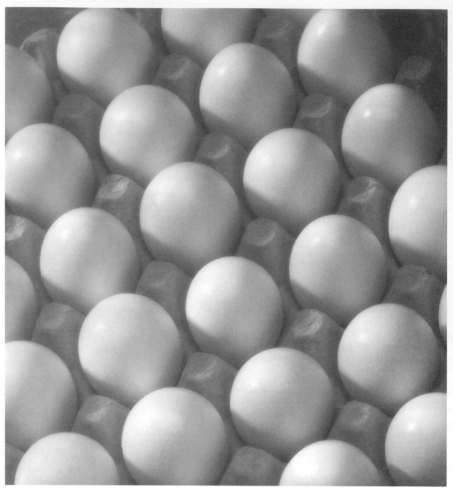

Eggs are similar to meat in that they are also a rich source of protein.

1995, a dietitian from the University of Washington summarized a study of 141 volunteers by saying that two eggs a day will not hurt you if you avoid the bacon that is usually served with the eggs. Three months after the test group had eaten two eggs a day, their cholesterol levels had changed, on average, from 227 to 233, which is insignificant. Half the volunteers actually increased their levels of good cholesterol.[40]

Of course, we should eat eggs only from clean fowl, not buzzards or other scavenger birds, or the eggs of serpents. The prophet likened wicked people to unclean snakes when he said:

They hatch the eggs of vipers and spin a spider's web. Whoever eats their eggs will die, and when one is broken, an adder is hatched (Isa. 59:5).

My conclusion is that eggs are much less harmful to human vascular systems than many medical scientists have previously believed. A study done by the American Cancer Society on 800,000 people showed that eggs protected against heart attack and strokes.[41] As we have seen, the yoke contains various beneficial enzymes such as lecithin, as well as vitamins and minerals. These ingredients apparently allow us to utilize the cholesterol in the yoke in a healthful way. The most nutritious eggs come from free-range chickens, not from the commercially fed chickens.

Meats in Conclusion

Oh—about that football game in which my opponent and I were playing erratically.

Colorado's coaches had developed plans that called on 35 to 40 players to carry out specific and complex

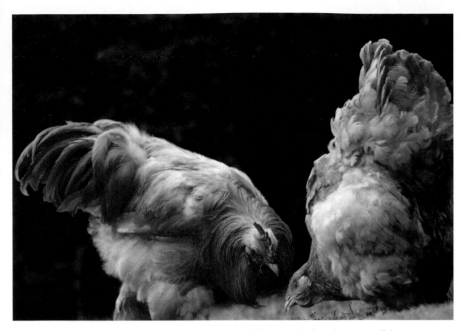

Eat the flesh of organically raised and chemical-free animals when possible.

tasks. The plans were good, and their players had more than enough skill to carry out the job. Colorado had great difficulty during that game because one very skilled behemoth did not obey his coaches' game plan and allowed me—his opponent—to mess up some of his team's carefully crafted plays.

Likewise, God has carefully developed a plan and a genetic design that will protect us from many opponents of our health. He has given us a well-designed plan that includes meats, and we have the ability to carry out that plan. But if we allow the opponents of good health to invade—if we don't block them out—they will destroy God's plan for our health.

First you need to study God's plan for your health. Then you need to put that plan into action by using discipline and enthusiasm. You may not succeed on every play—no player or team ever does. But if you give it the "good old college try," you will thrive.

In Summary

Consider meat a celebration or luxury food. You do not need much—4 ounces a day will supply what you need for protein. If you are concerned about getting enough protein, remember that your protein needs may be supplied by plant foods as well.

Eat only clean flesh, distinguishing between the clean and the unclean (see Lev. 11:46).

Eat the flesh of organically raised and chemical-free animals when possible.

Enjoy unprocessed and unpacked meats from cow, sheep, goats, deer and antelope; as well as chicken, quail and other game birds, and swimming fish that have both fins and scales, as listed in the Bible.

Low-fat beef, such as that from longhorns and Jersey breeds, or chickens, raised without chemicals and growth stimulants, are a treasure worth buying and eating. It is worth searching for the treat of eggs from free-range chickens.

Meats to avoid include hot dogs, sausages, lunch meats and cold cuts. In my opinion, hot dogs fall into the category of "trashy-rancid" meats. Often these kinds of meat are made of waste products and contain 50 percent fat. (Not to mention an FDA requirement that forbids hot dogs from including more than 20 percent animal hair.)

Avoid commercial gelatins made from pork and horse meat and containing color additives and chemicals along with mostly sugar and water.

Avoid ham, bacon and pork of any kind. Avoid catfish, shellfish and other toxic beasts.

Don't become addicted to (i.e., worship) meat. It is not necessary to have it at every meal or even every day. Two or three times a week is plenty.

Ingest no fats or blood.

Maybe it's time to get off our rump roast and eat more of everything God created for food.

9. How Sweet It Is

Many wonderfully designed foods taste sweet. It's as though God took the very best He had for humans and laced them with natural sugars.

Once when I was looking for something to drink at a convenience store, a three-year-old girl was begging her grandfather for some bottled water (what a smart little girl). Her grandfather said, "Honey, let me get you a red soda pop and not waste my money on water."

No, no—give her water, that's what's best for her, I thought. It was as though the little girl knew this Scripture verse that unexpectedly came into my mind:

I have more insight than all my teachers, . . . I have more understanding than the elders, for I obey your precepts
(Ps. 119:99,100).

Youth versus experience; wisdom verses folly. Who would win? Granddad won. He bought two red soda pops for his granddaughter.

What could be wrong with sugar? Sugar is organic and natural! It is low in calories. Sugar is a carbohydrate; it only has four calories per gram. If it isn't good for us, why was sugar created?

Are any sweeteners good?

We are told that some healthy people consume 80 percent of their calories in the form of carbohydrates. Other healthy people eat as little as 20 percent.

Regarding carbohydrates, Dr. Atkins recommends eating almost no carbohydrates to maintain proper weight and to lose fat.[1] On the other hand, Dr. Pritikin endorses a diet high in carbohydrates.[2] The advice goes on and on.

The Three Principles we are following in this book would insist that if we (1) eat sugars in the items God created for food, (2) before they are changed into toxic products and (3) if we don't get addicted to them, we are using sugars in healthful ways.

Some Sweet Definitions

What are carbohydrates, sugars and starches anyway? How are they related to proteins and fats? First, let's define a few terms before we get into the "sweet" of this chapter.

"Organic" is the term used to describe any nutrient that is present in living things. Organic compounds include the essentials of life, that is: amino acids, fatty acids and carbohydrates.

Chemically, carbon is the cornerstone element of all organic compounds. The carbon atom has four connectors (bonds) or electrons. When hooked together like boxcars, two of the four bonds are hooked to adjacent carbon atoms, leaving two other bonds free. If the two remaining bonds are hooked to water (H_2O), it is a simple carbohydrate (sugar; carbo- from carbon and hydrate from water).

If hydrogen instead of water (H_2O) is hooked to the carbon chain, a fatty acid is formed.

If ammonia is hooked to the carbon chain, it is an amino acid rather than a fatty acid or carbohydrate.

Simple carbohydrates have three to seven carbon atoms hooked together. Five or six carbons in a chain are the nutritionally important sugars utilized by our cells. They are called *monosaccharides* (MS). Some familiar names in this category include glucose, fructose and galactose.

Two MSs hooked together are called *disaccharides* (DS). Both mono- and disaccharides are called simple sugars. When several simple sugars are hooked together they are starches or polysaccharides. The structure of these starches is very important. (Complex carbohydrates [starches] are found in grains, legumes, nuts, fruits and vegetables. In this chapter we will learn how to use simple sugars in your diet.)

Purpose, Pattern and Design

Our cells have enzymes that have specific patterns that allow us to break the starch molecules into glucose, which is utilized for energy.

Cellulose and hemicellulose are also glucose molecules hooked together, but in a different configuration. Our enzyme system is not equipped to digest them. A lot of useless carbohydrates appear to be present in the things God created for food.

Did God really waste these carbohydrates? Did He mess up? No, and here is why.

Cellulose is insoluble fiber, and hemicellulose is soluble fiber. God, thank You for not giving us that one extra enzyme. If we digested the fiber out of our food we would all suffer from varicose veins, diverticula, hypoglycemia, hemorrhoids, constipation, gallstones, hiatal hernia, diabetes, peptic ulcers or appendicitis.

Remember that amino acids occur as mirror images as do the left and right hand. Sugars do also. Anything living has only left-handed amino acids and only right-handed simple carbohydrates.

The mirror image molecules are toxic to all life. Random chance would select 50 percent left and 50 percent right of these mirror images in constructing either proteins or carbo-

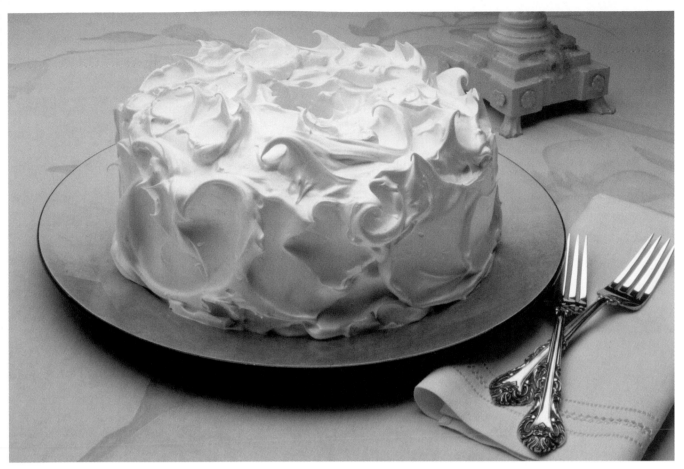

Many wonderfully designed foods taste sweet. It's as though God took the very best He had and laced them with natural sugars.

hydrates—and there would be no life. It is the same old story—random chance has no chance.

Glucose is the single simple sugar carried to our cells by the blood for energy. Glucose is necessary for the cells to connect amino acids, which build proteins (enzymes, hormones, etc.).

Glucose is also necessary for fat metabolism. If glucose is not available, the body mobilizes fat or proteins to supply the cells' need for energy. If the blood glucose levels are high, the glucose forms fat in our bodies.

The simple carbohydrate glucose is essential for the function and vitality of nerve tissue. If the glucose levels are low, the nerves will not function, causing irritability and eventually unconsciousness and death.

One by-product of glucose metabolism is *glucuronic acid,* which combines with toxic chemicals and bacterial toxins in our blood. The body excretes all these toxins with our bile.

How convenient! Blind luck again?

Many B vitamins are utilized in this process. Simple sugars require B-vitamins to be digested and metabolized. All carbohydrate-rich foods have an abundance of B-vitamins so the body can assimilate them well.

What happens when we process sugar, thus removing the B-vitamins? The body has to supply them from other sources.

In *Sugar Blues,* William Dufty tells of a shipwreck. The ship's cargo contained refined sugar. The survivors were marooned on an island. The sailors ate sugar and water only for the nine days they were stranded. Their rescuers found them in a wasted and toxic condition.

Many fasting experiments have shown that health improves with a water-only diet for up to 21 days or longer. The marooned sailors' surprisingly poor health can be attributed to severe vitamin deficiencies caused by the toxic effects of sugar. The sugar depleted the available B-vitamins previously ingested with recent meals. It does the same in our bodies.

Many wonderfully designed foods taste sweet. It is as though God took the very best He had for humans and laced them with natural sugars and complex carbohydrates.

When God designed our tongue, God created taste buds. One of four kinds of taste buds was specifically blueprinted to appreciate the wonder of the sweet flavor.

Just as a hummingbird is attracted to sweet syrup, so humans are pleased with sweet things. The Latin word *frui,* which gives us our word "fruit," means "enjoy." If eaten in their natural states, the sweet flavors of fruits and vegetables are good for you because they contain fiber and other essential nutrients.

These natural "sweet foods" also contain many protective ingredients that help prevent and fight off illnesses.

In previous chapters we discovered that proteins and fats seemed to be purposefully designed. Now we see that carbohydrates also appear to be carefully designed.

Sweets and Principle I

Do you suppose there is a Designer?

I believe there is, and that He took great care in His Design to keep my mind and body healthy by using the food He created. And the sweets He created are some of the most enjoyable of all foods.

The Gift of Honey

One of the God-designed sweets is honey. If this delightful stuff is mentioned 56 times in the King James Version of the Bible, surely it is a sweetener that has been created for food.

Honey is mentioned in an Old Testament Messianic prophecy:

Therefore the Lord himself shall give you a sign; Behold a virgin shall conceive, and bear a son, and shall call his name Immanuel. Butter and honey shall he eat, that he may know to refuse the evil, and choose the good (Isa. 7:14,15, KJV).

Sanctioned as it is by the prophet's prediction of Jesus—the Messiah—we are certainly to assume that honey is intended to be food for us. After all, if Jesus and John the Baptist ate it, it's good enough for me!

Let's look at some more passages that confirm from Scripture that honey was created for food.

After Jesus had risen from the dead, He appeared to His disciples.

And they gave him a piece of a broiled fish, and of an honeycomb (Luke 24:42, KJV).

Some scholars speculate that Jesus may have deliberately eaten in front of the disciples after His resurrection to counteract a heresy maintaining that the flesh is evil, and that Jesus, being divine, could not have a real, flesh-and-blood body that could eat real food. By eating fish and honey, Jesus once and for all overcame that heresy.

In nearly all references to honey, it is mentioned in a positive connotation. For example:

My son, eat thou honey, because it is good; and the honeycomb, which is sweet to thy taste (Prov. 24:13, KJV).

Some think that honey is great for our health.[3] On the other hand, some health professionals say honey in the diet makes little difference. I had a conversation with a physician who owns one of the largest honey suppliers in our country. He maintained that there was no difference between his honey and sugar.

Another study indicated many differences between honey and refined sugar. Researchers found 165 ingredients in honey, very few of which are found in sugar.[4] They were unable to determine all the functions of these associated food factors contained in honey. We do know, however, that honey contains various enzymes, minerals, amino acids and vitamins that aid in digestion. Also, the biblical references to the fact that honey provides good nourishment are difficult to refute.

Many challenge studies have pointed to the superior value of raw honey as compared to dextrose sugar and other sugars. Diabetics can sometimes tolerate honey better than refined sugars. Honey certainly has more nutritional value than other sugar-packed products; it is also absorbed more slowly than sugar.

We should note, however, that honey also has a substance in it that causes nausea if too much is eaten. This ingredient probably prevents "spikes" or abrupt elevations in blood glucose from overeating.

Scripture provided this warning all along:

Hast thou found honey? eat so much as is sufficient for thee, lest thou be filled therewith, and vomit it (Prov. 25:16, KJV).

Did Solomon speak from personal experience, perhaps having come upon some honey and eaten too much when he was a shepherd boy? Or was he a biochemist? Or was he just divinely inspired?

Scripture leaves no doubt about the health value of honey:

Pleasant words are as an honeycomb, sweet to the soul, and health to the bones (Prov. 16:24, KJV).

Honey contains 18 amino acids, each helpful to humans. Proline, an amino acid that is most highly concentrated in honey, is the primary component in collagen. Collagen is the main structure in bone. Read Proverbs 16:24 one more time.

Calcium is found in two forms in honey. Eleven other valuable minerals are also present.

Should we eat the honeycomb or the honey? Honey freed from the comb or heated loses its amino acids, including proline—which remains as long as the honey is in the comb.

The high osmolarity of honey—its ability to permeate cell membranes—enables it to kill bacteria and other germs by pulling all fluids through the cell membranes. In addition, some natural antibiotics in honey work as an effective element in cleaning infected open wounds.

When bees are collecting nectar from plants, the chemical sprays that may be present on the plants are not transferred to the honey. I don't understand how they avoid those chemicals. The nectar is digested by the bee, and the chemicals are apparently detoxified before the honey is excreted. We still should not eat too much honey, particularly if we know that it comes from heavily sprayed fields.

Have you ever studied a beehive? In that first-ever hive, many instincts had to be fully developed in those 75,000 bees for the hive to survive. The first queen could not have survived without a full component of skilled worker bees or drones. The hexagonal shape of the comb has been calculated by engineers to be the best design for storage and strength. Study the beehive and one more time you will say: "Random chance has no chance."

Sweeteners and Principle II

What about processed honey?

Raw or unheated honey in its comb is preferable. Some producers, such as the physician who reported that his honey was no different from sugar, heat and strain the honey to make it more liquid for bottling purposes. This heating destroys some of the valued properties in the honey. Long feeding a dry, sugary cereal to one group of rats. The box containing the cereal was fed to a similar group of rats. The study indicated that the rats who ate the box thrived better than those who ate the cereal.[6] This makes sense because the rats that were fed the box were essentially fasting, which is better than the rats eating toxic white flour, sugars (up to 60 percent in the cereal used) and artificial colors.

Parents would do well to try to keep children from becoming addicted to sugar-laced cereals. Most cereals targeted for children have three to five times more sugar and one-third of the fiber of other cereals.[7]

Aspartame Alert[8]

During a recent year, 80 percent of the complaints filed about food additives were pertaining to Aspartame, the sweetener in NutraSweet. Five deaths were reported. Symptoms included headaches, dizziness, balance problems, depression, vomiting, abdominal pain, diarrhea, altered vision, weakness, seizures, numbness, hives, memory loss and sleep disorders.

One of the components of Aspartame—aspartic acid—is a neurotoxin. Another component, phenylalanine, is considered harmful to the unborn, and facilitates seizures. A final component, wood alcohol, is a generalized toxin, particularly harmful to the brain and the eyes.

When heated or in liquid form, aspartame breaks down into products thought by some researchers to cause brain tumors.[9]

Aspartame reactions frequently reproduce symptoms similar to chronic fatigue syndrome, Alzheimer's Disease, epilepsy, multiple sclerosis, post-polio syndrome, carpal tunnel syndrome, Lyme Disease, myalgia, Lou Gehrig's Disease and anxiety phobia disorders.

In defense of Aspartame, sugar abuse can cause many of these same symptoms. Certainly these diseases are frequently caused by other factors. Aspartame sometimes mimics the symptoms of these diseases.

According to *The Food Additive Book*, research before Aspartame was released on the market in the United

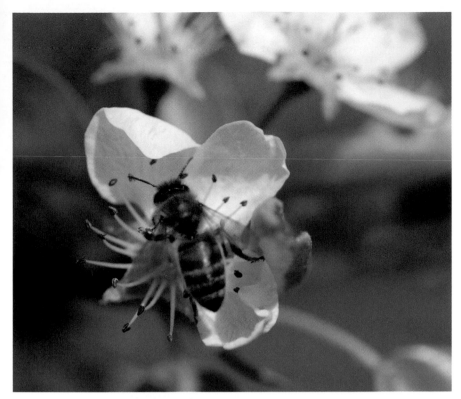

When bees are collecting nectar from plants, the chemical sprays that may be present on the plants are not transferred to the honey.

ago in the ancient writings of the Ayurvedic healers of India, heated honey was thought to be harmful.[5] I'm not sure what qualities are lost once it is heated, but certainly the enzymes could be denatured. I don't think much damage is done at proper cooking temperatures, but no research has been done to demonstrate either way.

An occasional case of severe infection in babies who were fed honey has been reported. No report has specified whether or not the honey had been processed, heated or denatured.

Honey is also sometimes strained to remove pollen and other ingredients. Pollen is loaded with nutrients. It is used as a supplement by many people. Honey is healthier when the pollen is not removed.

Other sweeteners mentioned in the Bible are freshly squeezed juices, dates and sugar cane. If these sugars are dehydrated at relatively low temperatures, many of their ingredients are preserved.

Today we have many other kinds of sweeteners. Based on The Three Principles, these sweeteners could be classified from best to worst placing honey at the top, followed in declin-

ing order by rice malt, barley malt, molasses, date sugar, fruit-juice sugars, maple syrup, beet sugar, corn syrup, cane sugar and—if you must—NutraSweet. It is my impression that most of the corn, cane and beet sugars are heavily processed, leaving them denatured, white and devitalized.

Barley and rice sweeteners are low in calories but very sweet. One advantage of barley and molasses is that they are not heavily processed. Processed maple syrup may be slightly better than other syrups. Molasses ranks higher nutritionally than raw sugars, but honey is still the best product. Turbinado sugar and brown sugar contain a little molasses for coloring, but are otherwise no different from white (naked) sugar.

The more commonly used sugars such as those from cane, beets and corn are more likely to increase allergic reactions. Therefore, I would avoid them as much as possible.

All of these sources are great in their natural state. By the time many of these sweeteners find their way to your table, they have often gone through 10 stages of processing. Does this make any difference?

A typical science project reports

States showed an increased incidence of brain cancer in rats that were fed aspartame.[10] Since 1981, the incidence of brain tumors has gradually increased. It remains nearly impossible to prove a one-to-one correlation, but many people have eradicated many strange symptoms by withdrawing from Aspartame.

Many of the symptoms and diseases mentioned are probably dose related. The biblical warning against too much is still applicable. It is my impression that both sugar and Aspartame are addictive. Many people consume much too much. People striving for good health should stay away from both sugar and artificial sweeteners as much as possible.

Artificial sweeteners and sugar stimulate hunger. Someone trying to lose weight and eating artificial sweeteners or sugar will probably consume more food because of the craving caused by these sweeteners. People trying to gain weight might be well advised to drink diet sodas before meals to stimulate their appetite.

Other names of sugars to be avoided include sucrose, dextrose, fructose, lactose, dextrin, maltose, monosaccharides and disaccharides, and syrup. Here is one of the most unusual names for a sugar: *unbleached evaporated cane juice crystals*. That one was found on a commercial cookie. Know what it means? Sugar!

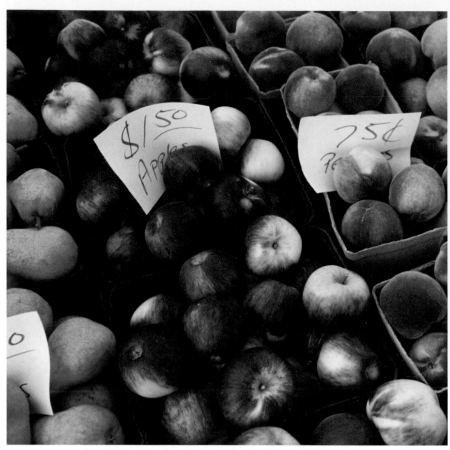

One candy bar has the same amount of sugar as 10 apples.

Sweeteners and Principle III

The idea here (which can be applied to all foods) is that natural sweets themselves are not bad, but they should be controlled in quantity and quality so they can truly be enjoyed. We need to avoid overindulging, including on natural sweets. Remember what the wise man said:

It is not good to eat too much honey (Prov. 25:27).

One tablespoon of honey supplies the nutritional value of one piece of fruit. The body can digest and utilize one or two pieces of fruit or two tablespoons of honey in an hour. One candy bar has the same amount of sugar as 10 apples.

Do you heed the advice to be moderate in your sugar intake? Do you think eating six feet of sugar cane every day would be too much? How much is too much? I don't know. Surely everyone has different limits, because we are all unique.

In the United States, sugar intake has increased from 1 percent to 20 percent of total calories during the last 200 years. An interesting statistic is that during that time frame our fat intake has not changed.

The average American consumes 150 pounds of refined sugar a year in this country.[11] Some people eat as much as 350 pounds of sugar a year—one pound a day. If we ate sugar cane prior to processing, we would receive many of the essentials needed for life, in addition to large amounts of fiber. Processing takes away the nutrients, however, and what remains is "pure, refined, white sugar" (naked calories) that has little benefit and can be detrimental to human health.

Is sugar killing your "sweetie"? Probably.

Does your "honey" have crooked teeth, obesity, frequent infections, allergies, hyperactivity, dyslexia, depression, addictions and blood clots? Sugar probably contributes to these problems.[12]

Dr. John Yudkin and others agree that sweets, rather than fats, increase the risk of heart attacks. Diets high in sugar elevate cholesterol and triglycerides, making sugar as risky as smoking or obesity.[13] Other studies show that VLDL (bad) cholesterol can be lowered by a diet low in simple sugar.

In one study, heart patients were found to eat 128 grams of sugar a day, and a comparable group of healthy people ate only 58 grams of sugar a day. The fat consumption of both groups, however, was the same.

Similar studies show the same cause-and-effect relationship for gallstones, colon cancer, appendicitis, ulcers, chronic fatigue syndrome and immune disorder.

Are you getting the idea that people generally eat too much sugar?

The food industry knows that people become addicted to sugars. Sugar creates product loyalty. Heavy concentrations of these sugars are found in beverages, jams, preserves, cookies, cakes, pies, pastries, donuts, ice milk, sherbets, sugared gelatin, canned fruits, canned juices, Kool-Aid, sodas, candy, chocolate and chewing gum. It might surprise you to know that sugar is added to small salt packets, cans of vegetables, catsup and salad dressings. A tomato sauce cannot be sold as "catsup" if it is not sugared.

When I was visiting a friend in the hospital I took special interest in his diabetic food tray. I noticed a "no sugar added" milk drink and was interested because I am a diabetic, too. To my surprise, the label included dextrin, monosaccharide, disaccharide and corn syrup. This label includes four simple sugars. This drink probably contained more sugar than milk. My diabetic friend really liked his drink! It is not easy to avoid sugars, but it is a great idea.

Enjoy honey, fruit juices, barley sweetener and black strap molasses. One tablespoon of honey is equivalent in sweetness to five tablespoons of sugar. When cooking with honey, reduce the total amount of other liquids by one-quarter cup, per cup of honey.[14] Also, lower the baking temperature 50 degrees to prevent over-baking.

Enjoy the things created for food that contain natural sugars. Enjoy complex carbohydrates.

If you must eat sugar, make sure you eat plenty of fiber and nutrients along with it.

Peanut Butter Candy

1 cup natural peanut butter
(*It's a great treasure hunt in the maze of your local grocery store to find some without added sugar.*)
1/2 cup honey (may use 1/4 cup)
1/2 cup nonfat dry milk
3 T. toasted wheat germ
Mix ingredients. Press into buttered dish, chill and cut into cubes. This mixture can be rolled, chilled and sliced.

Peach Pie

5 or 6 good-size peaches. Peel and slice
1/2 cup honey
1 T. quick-cooking tapioca
Line pie pan with whole-grain pastry. Fill with sliced peaches. Sprinkle with tapioca. Pour honey over peaches. Cover with strips of pastry. Bake 40 minutes at 425°.

Many simple recipes are available. Experiment!

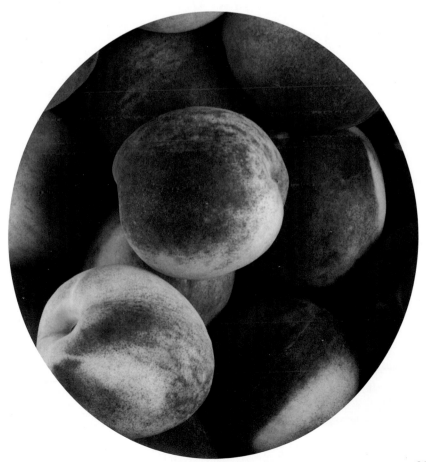

10. Mom Was Right: Eat your Fruits and Veggies

As Daniel and his friends learned in Babylonian captivity . . .

Super, awesome, colossal, wonderful, cool, fantastic!

Descriptions of a great running back for the NFL? Maybe.

Descriptions of a new movie? Possibly.

Descriptions of a gorgeous sunset? Could be.

Descriptions of vegetables and fruits and what they can do for your body? Positively!

This is a great topic to write about because it has no "avoid" lists. It has only "eat all and more than you could possibly think of eating" lists.

Definitions: Technical and Common

What are vegetables? Some say the vegetable kingdom is the entire world of plants; but let's get more specific.

According to another meaning, the term "vegetable" refers to foods we obtain from the leaves, stems, flower clusters, roots, tubers (underground stems), seeds or fruits of plants.

Technically, then cucumbers, eggplants, peppers, squashes, tomatoes and string beans—all of which are commonly called vegetables—are fruits.

That's interesting, but for our purposes let's just call vegetables and fruits what we commonly call them. Fruits include apples, bananas, grapes, oranges, peaches, pears, strawberries and so on.

Vegetables include cabbage, lettuce, spinach, asparagus, potatoes, carrots, beets, corn and so on.

Both definitions are sometimes appropriate in this chapter.

Chock-Full of Benefits

Fruits and vegetables comprise a large group of foods that humans can enjoy. When God first created this world, these foods flourished in the beautiful Garden of Eden. These first foods continue to provide outstanding nourishment, and they can be enjoyed in their natural state with very little risk.

Fruits and veggies come loaded with complex carbohydrates and other essentials for life, such as amino acids and essential fatty acids. They also include many of the natural vitamins and minerals vital to human nutrition.

Additionally, these products have literally thousands of other phytochemicals briefly discussed in earlier chapters. Fruits and vegetables also have both soluble and insoluble fiber that allows our bodies to select what nutrients are needed. This fiber allows many unneeded calories to pass through the intestinal tract.

Conventional wisdom has indicated that eating vegetables alone will result in humans becoming deficient in proteins, minerals and vitamins. Studies of people living on vegetables, fruits, berries and nuts, however, indicate that this conclusion lacks accuracy. Admittedly, some dangers are to be avoided by vegetarians. They would be at greater risk, for example, if they ate processed fruits, grains and vegetables. Processing can destroy much of the nutrient package created in our foods, thus violating our Principle II.

Preventable Diseases

Many studies have shown that if we ate our veggies, as Mom told us, along with more fruit as well, we could avoid or cure several common ailments.

Obesity

In 1970, Dr. Dennis Burkett's study at a military base in Africa confirmed the benefits of eating high-fiber foods such as fruits and vegetables. Native prisoners were compared to a group of soldiers. The natives who were studied ate vegetables, grains and breads they had grown. The military personnel ate processed sugars, white bread and other refined foods. Both groups ate the same number of calories a day. Fecal material from each of the participants was collected for several days.

The caloric content of the fecal material of the military personnel contained 20 percent of the ingested calories. In contrast, the feces of the natives contained 60 percent of the caloric content of what they had eaten.

This increased absorption of calories from refined foods underscores why so many people who do not get enough fiber from foods such as fruits and vegetables become obese.[1]

Bad Cholesterol, or Triglycerides

Studies have revealed excellent results in preventing heart disease and in reducing the damaging type of lipids (triglycerides, or so-called "bad cholesterol") in the blood by eating garlic, carrots and corn. Oats, barley,

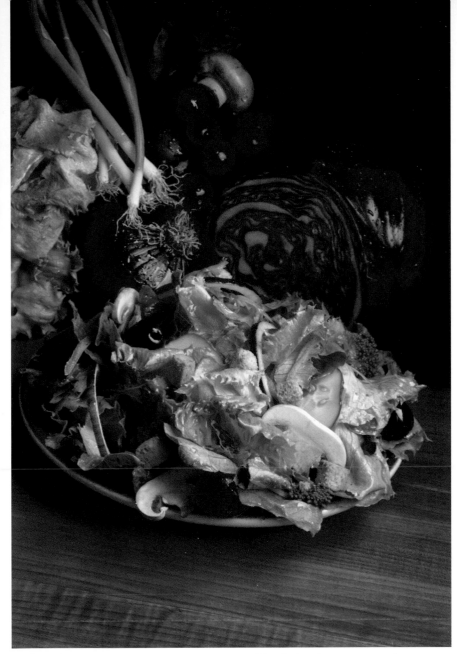

Fruits and vegetables comprise a large group of foods that humans can enjoy.

recovery was complete within a few months. The only thing that caused her symptoms to recur was when she began adding processed foods and meats to her diet, so she soon dropped those foods. She was the belle of the ball at the reunion; and she has remained healthy for the 18 years since.

Cancer

In the big picture, eating fruits and vegetables is more beneficial than taking vitamins because the foods give you a broad spectrum of synergistic nutrients.

Let's just think about eating carrots as opposed to taking an over-the-counter vitamin pill—beta-carotene. Carrots contain thousands of nutrients, including more than 200 types of carotene. When you take a beta-carotene vitamin pill, you are taking only part of the spectrum. As you can see, research projects that study only one isolated nutrient may be confusing.

Eating fruits and vegetables has been shown to decrease cancer of the lung in smokers. Every day for four years, 29,000 Finnish smokers were given either a dummy pill, a supplement of beta-carotene or a vitamin E pill. To the surprise of the research team, the carotene increased the cancer risk by 18 percent. The carotene supplement contained only one type of carotene. Compare this to a Genesis 1:29 diet (essentially vegetarian), which would have hundreds of different types of beta-carotenes![3]

Other cancer research reminds us of Principle II: Eat created food before it is changed into nutrient-deficient or toxic substances, and before its individual nutrients have been isolated by processing. Any single nutrient by itself may be good or it may be toxic.

In one study, vitamin C, beta-carotene and vitamin E or a placebo were given during a four year period to 751 people who had previous colon tumors.[4] These nutrients were chosen because they are highly concentrated in fruits and vegetables that clearly protect against colon tumors. These three nutrients are also known to be strong antioxidants, which appear to be the active ingredients in fruits and vegetables that prevent tumors.

lemongrass, rice, tea, sprouts, exercise and low-fat beef (six ounces a day) were also effective.[2]

Collagen (Connective Tissue) Disease

A young mother in Dallas had scleroderma—a disease that affects the blood vessels and connecting tissue, often making the skin excessively firm or even hard. She was also bedridden with deforming arthritis. Her physician, who was also her employer, thought she was terminally ill. Her mother was taking care of her and her children. Unwilling to give up, the patient started reading everything

available from anywhere, and gradually accumulated a notebook of suggestions she thought were appropriate for her problem.

Basically, she started on a diet consisting mainly of vegetable broth. Later she started eating whole-grain, sugarless bran muffins. I saw her several months later at our twentieth high school reunion. I had heard she was terminally ill, but there she was—dancing with, talking to, hugging and smiling at everyone.

What happened? I just had to know what she had done to be looking so good. She explained that after six to eight days of eating her unusual broth she started feeling much better. Her

To the surprise of the authors, no difference was noted between the two groups. The study concluded that "it looks like the best approach right now is to eat whole foods." In my opinion, the whole nutrient package in a food is superior to any of its parts.

Those in the groups who had previously eaten plenty of fruits and vegetables, however, still showed evidence of protection. Apparently many other ingredients in fruits and vegetables are present that make these antioxidants more effective. Thousands of ingredients called "unknown food factors" require precise concentrations for the food's nutrients to be maximally bioavailable for our bodies.

How did the food factors get there? Choose one answer:

1. Random chance—luck. (That would be like expecting a tornado hitting an alphabet-soup factory to write the dictionary.)

2. The fruits and veggies themselves made unknown food factors to protect us. (Praise the Apricot? Thank you, mighty Plum? Indwell me, holy Carrot?)

3. A magnificent design. (Thank You, Perfect and Awesome Creator, for providing for our needs in the things You designed for food.)

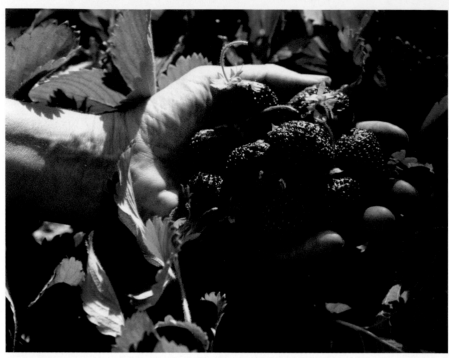

Eating fruits and vegetables is the place to start for illness prevention and recovery.

Health from Genesis 1

I read many newsletters and summaries of newsletters about health. The experts in nutrition for each disease process give a lot of advice. Some of it is bizarre, but most seem to agree that eating fruits and vegetables is the place to start for both prevention and recovery. Again, this is the stuff of Genesis 1:29:

Then God said, "I give you every seed-bearing plant on the face of the whole earth and every tree that has fruit with seed in it. They will be yours for food."

Dr. Albert Anderson, an allergist, encourages his patients to eat organic food that is unprocessed, scavenger free and so on. He told me that it soon became obvious which patients followed "The" diet. He "lost" those

patients to good health, but he gained their friendship.

Principle I, eating that which God created for food; and Principle II, eating these foods as fresh and unprocessed as possible, remain very important.

No wonder Paul could use fruit for a spiritual analogy:

Being filled with the fruits [author's emphasis] *of righteousness, which are by Jesus Christ, unto the glory and praise of God* (Phil. 1:11, KJV).

Doing things right (righteousness), and appropriating the righteousness of Christ yield fruits that are glorious and praiseworthy to God.

May I extrapolate from this spiritual truth to say that fruits that are grown right deserve glory and praise to God for providing us such extraordinary foods?

In a perfect world, we would daily pick and eat food from our own gardens, as Adam and Eve did in Genesis 1 in their Garden of Eden. The soil would be rich and chemical free.

Although the world is not perfect, we must not use that as an excuse to neglect to provide our bodies with the health available through fruits and vegetables. Adam's "the-woman-thou-gavest-me" excuse does not

work either. Working and sweating to raise a garden or to locate these God-given foods is worth your effort.

And sow the fields, and plant vineyards, which may yield fruits of increase (Ps. 107:37, KJV).

Work hard at this, whether sowing and reaping or buying your fruits and veggies. Don't be a fool, however, and think you have too much to do to take time to rest. Even God's work gets done better if you take off one day a week.

"Six days do your work, but on the seventh day do not work, so that your ox and your donkey may rest and the slave born in your household, and the alien as well, may be refreshed" (Exod. 23:12).

Fasting helps, too (see chapter 5).

Once you have located food, eat it. The longer the storage time, the greater the loss of nutrients. Although, as in the case of grains, God has designed protection for the nutrients in fruits and vegetables, the fresher they are, the better. Vitamin C is lost the quickest, but many other important nutrients remain. Even dried fruits have many good nutrients left.

Cooking releases some nutrients from the Designer's "packets" in which fruits and veggies store their nutritious treasures. Although heat actually makes them more bioavailable, they begin to deteriorate fairly quickly. A rating of the most nourishing forms of fruits and vegetables, including ways to prepare them, looks like this: (1) raw, (2) steamed, (3) baked, (4) soups or broth, (5) freshly squeezed juice, (6) frozen, (7) stir-fried, (8) canned . . . and (25!) deep-fried.

The Way to Healthier, Wiser Kids

The lifestyles of the young Hebrew Daniel and his friends provide great examples of the healthful qualities of vegetables, and of eating according to God's Law. Their story is told in the first chapter of Daniel.

As you may recall, Daniel and his friends had been carried into Babylonian captivity; but they found favor with the king, and he selected them to serve in the palace. To prepare them, they were to be served royal food and wine, and trained for three years.

Daniel, however, determined to continue to eat according to God's Law. He asked for, and received, permission to eat only vegetables and water. After a 10-day test, if he and his friends did not fare better than others who ate and drank from the king's menu, the king's servants could treat them as he wished. Sure enough:

At the end of the ten days they looked healthier and better nourished than any of the young men who ate the royal food. In every matter of wisdom and understanding about which the king questioned them, he found them ten times better than all the magicians and enchanters in his whole kingdom (Dan. 1:15,20).

Yes, I am suggesting that you try this kind of dietary training not only on your own kids, but also on everyone in your family. It is a discipline that will benefit anyone who tries it.

Vegetables such as those Daniel and the three other Hebrews ate contain many bonus nutrients once called "associated food factors." Many have been researched recently. Associated food factors have been shown to protect humans from vascular disease, bacterial infections, viral infections, cancer and so on. The *Journal of the American Dietetics Association* states:

Never before has the focus on the health benefits of commonly available foods been so strong. The philosophy that food can be health promoting beyond its nutritional value is gaining acceptance in the scientific community as mounting research links diet/food components to disease prevention and treatment.[5]

This means that the total effect of the combined associated food factors and other nutrients has a greater effect when blended together than if the nutrients are isolated and used individually. Often these same isolated nutrients have little or no effect by themselves. Here again, the total package of nutrients in any of these foods listed in Genesis 1:29 is greater than the sum of its parts.

Fruits, Veggies and Principle II

The wise man said:

There is a way that seems right to a man, but in the end it leads to death (Prov. 14:12).

It also "seems right" to "civilized" man to violate Principle II by subjecting fresh fruits and vegetables to pro-

Try a fruit and vegetable diet on your own kids—and everyone else in your family.

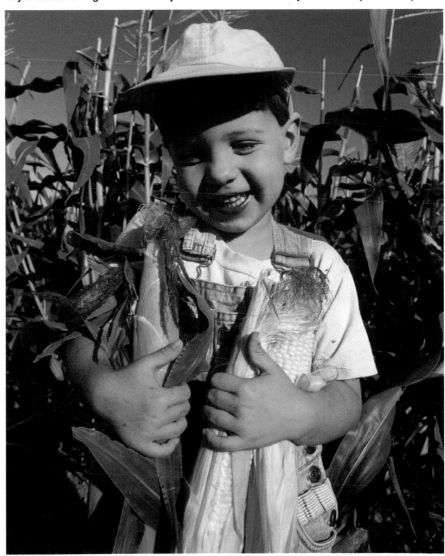

cessing, additives, sprays, chemical fertilizers and preservatives.

More than 8,000 chemicals are approved by the Food and Drug Administration for use in food. A few are healthy, but many can be very harmful. Good foods can negate many of the harmful effects of additives and processing; but for those who are serious about maintaining their health, organic, chemical-free foods are a real bargain at any price. Buying organic when possible is a way of staying away from unhealthful chemicals.

Dried fruit is processed minimally by the sun or hot air. The water content of such fruit is reduced from 80 percent to 20 percent. Water is present in fruit in a highly filtered form because it has passed from the soil through the stem and leaves of the plant. Dried fruit has a high concentration of minerals (iron, copper and potassium), fiber and beta-carotene. Be aware that dried fruit has as high as 70 percent fructose sugar, and that vitamin C is lost in the dehydrating process. If you eat a large amount of dried fruit, you may ingest too much in the way of simple sugars.

Other "Thorns and Thistles"

Sulfites (sulfur dioxide) are often added to retard color changes in fruits and vegetables. This substance keeps potatoes white and lettuce green.[6]

Sulfites are dangerous for millions of Americans who have allergies, particularly asthma. Symptoms include severe headaches, abdominal pains, facial flushing, diarrhea and faintness. Sulfite test strips for testing foods before you eat them can be purchased at a pharmacy.

Sulfites are used on most kinds of lettuce, keeping the greens fresh looking for a considerable time. Other foods that have added sulfites are baked products such as cookies; beverages (beer, wine, colas); desserts and other sugar-laden products; and fermented, frozen, fresh or canned vegetables or fruits.

I hope you are not sensitive to sulfites, but enough people are that many products are now produced without them. Ask for foods without them when you eat out. It would be better to pick wilted salad containing

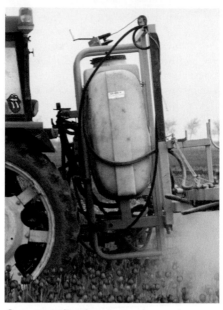
Crop-spraying on a farm.

no sulfites than to choose crisp greens containing sulfites.

Monosodium glutamate (MSG) is similar to sulfites, and according to some studies is toxic to many people. It is usually found in soups, Chinese foods and many other prepared foods.

I once entered a large chili cook-off. Before the tasting, I wandered back into the kitchen, and to my surprise, a lady was pouring MSG from a gallon jug into the various pots of chili.

"Why are you doing that?" I asked curiously.

"To make it taste good," was the reply. It is one of those myths that many are convinced is true. My chili placed second. I wonder if she sprinkled it, too. I don't think so.

Many people reportedly feel awful after consuming MSG.

Humans can lose their health by ignoring Principle II. Carefully guard against eating chemical additives and processed nutrient-deficient provisions.

Chemical sprays and even natural chemicals in vegetables can be toxic by overindulging. For example, apples treated by the chemical "alar" at doses that kill bugs can also be toxic to humans. It is probably better to share your apple with a worm than to eat an apple in which a worm can't live.

Worms also refuse to eat white sugar. They probably get a belly ache. Many of you do!

Maybe we need to be worm wise.

Worms will not eat chemicalized fruits or vegetables. Worm wisdom might pay dividends in health.

Watermelons, which in their natural state are a great food, have caused poisoning deaths when they were sprayed with a chemical to control pests. Reportedly, six people died from eating watermelon sprayed with pesticide.[7] It would seem wiser to let the bugs eat some, too, rather than to poison ourselves.

We could tell thousands of similar stories involving chemicals that have been added to food.

What about those who handle these pesticides? Farmers probably have the shortest life span of any profession.

Wise people seek organically grown, or at least chemical-free foods. Research is showing that chemical-free fruits, vegetables and nuts are treasures in protecting us from all diseases.

Revisiting Principle III

Principle III—avoiding addictions—also applies to these nutritious and tasty foods. Variety remains an important consideration even in the case of the treasure of fruits and veggies.

Idolatry That Can Kill

This is pretty simple. Don't worship a carrot, an apple or a turnip. Just thank God for them. It is impossible for me to judge whether someone is doing this. Some who are simply awestruck by the design of barley, carrots, squash, okra, banana and so on may become ambassadors for spreading the food's benefits to thousands. More power to them.

Avoiding addictions also applies to fruits and vegetables. Some people get "weird" and overindulge on one vegetable or fruit.

Some people eat only oranges, others just lettuce.

One patient came to my office with what was at first thought to be "yellow jaundice," but turned out to be carrotemia. The patient's skin had turned yellow from ingesting huge

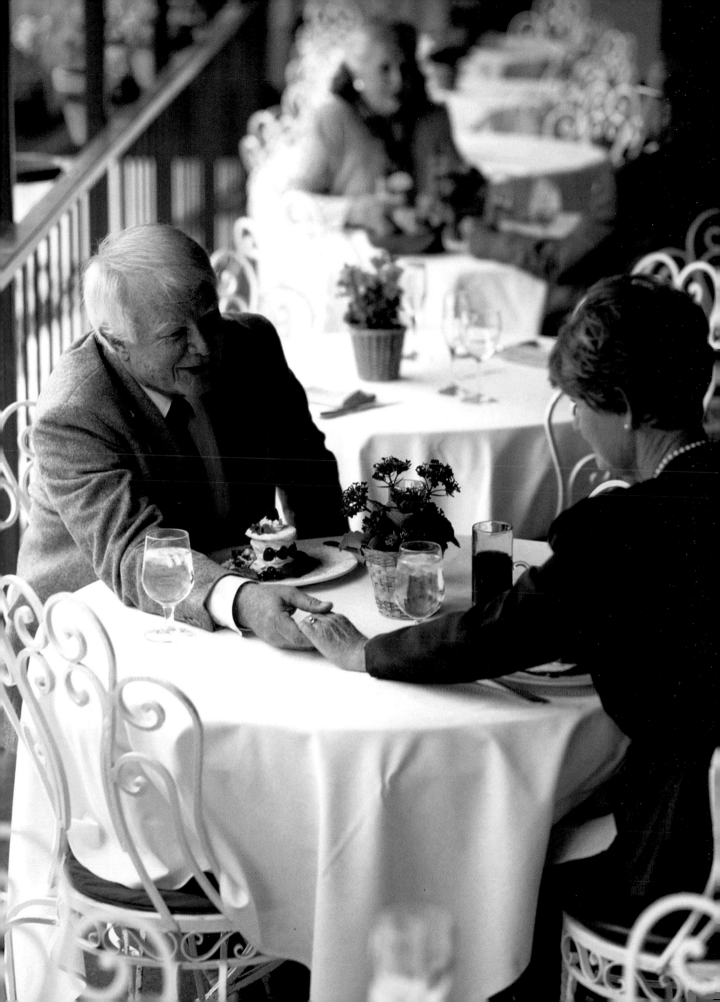

amounts of carrots or carrot juice. The pigment from the carrots had overwhelmed the normal skin color. No harm done. A few weeks fasting from carrots relieved the problem.

Broccoli can be toxic as well! Broccoli has the substance sulforaphane in it, which probably is the important chemical that acts as an antioxidant—and inhibits cancer. At certain concentrations, however, it is toxic. It will kill bugs—and damage your cells. Apparently the body has enzymes that metabolize this chemical satisfactorily; but these enzymes can be overwhelmed if huge amounts are eaten daily. (No chance, in my case; an enzyme is more likely to develop by random chance than I am likely to overeat on broccoli.)

Dr. James Marshall, an epidemiologist at State University of New York in Buffalo, has demonstrated that the protective effect of broccoli or any other vegetable is gained by eating combinations of vegetables rather than by eating any one type.[8]

What About Vegetarianism?

Jesus enjoyed and prepared meat, so I take it that no scriptural argument can be made against eating some meat. On the other hand, as we said earlier, the idea that eating only vegetables will result in deficiencies in proteins, minerals and vitamins is a myth. Although I am not a vegetarian, probably less than 5 percent of my calories come from meat.

Still, some dangers should be avoided by vegetarians. They will get into trouble if they eat only processed fruits, grains and vegetables. Processing destroys much of the nutrient package created in our foods. Another real danger in eating vegetables alone is the addition of chemical sprays and additives. Additives, hormones and pesticides remain active even after cooking and being digested.

Earl Mindell, a health writer, says this is particularly distressing because 2 billion pounds of highly toxic and potentially carcinogenic pesticides are used annually.[9]

The fiber and nutrients in vegetables do detoxify many of these additives. These nutrients, however, could be put to better use in the body if they were not wasted by these chemicals.

Recommendations

Eat to live, don't live to eat.

Be prepared to spend time, effort and money to find healthful fruits and veggies. Some use the excuse that it costs too much to eat right. A study reported in the *University of California-Berkeley Wellness Letter* showed that sicknesses in 40-year-old males at one company cost their employers $1,282 a year.[10] This was reduced by one half when the workers were able to change two or three obvious bad habits. If employees would learn to follow God's way and The Three Principles, the cost of their health care in most years would be zero.

Remember the one question we are asking and answering in this book is, "If a perfect God created us, why am I sick?" (see chapter 1).

Are you beginning to get the picture?

It's worth repeating: Eat to live, don't live to eat.

Vegetables should be included every day in your meals. The American Cancer Society recommends eating five to seven vegetables and fruits every day. Enjoy more.

Eat fresh vegetables soon after they have been peeled or cooked.

Cooked vegetables have the following advantages: heat breaks down enzyme inhibitors that prevent digestion of proteins in peanuts and beans. In the case of some fruits and vegetables, vitamin B1 and other nutrients can be made more bioavailable by heating. Also, cooking will destroy several toxic bacteria such as salmonella.

A word of caution involving fruits. For diabetics, the intake of fruits must be balanced against exercise and insulin. Fruit juices do include simple sugars that can tax the body's ability to maintain blood sugars at reasonable levels. In middle-eastern countries, juices are diluted with water in approximately a 4-1 ratio, and are still tasty and nutritious.

Enjoy the hundreds of varieties of vegetables and fruits available. I don't believe you can eat too many fresh or properly prepared vegetables.

Fruits and veggies offer the opportunity of fulfilling a fantasy: stuff yourself and lose weight.

11. The Spice(s) of Life

Spice up your life with some of the zestful herbs and seasonings a loving God has created.

If you had dropped by my father-in-law's house about 6:00 A.M. on any April Fool's Day, you could have heard him muttering something about, "They did it again!"

Although he always "bit," his daughters could be counted on regularly to put salt in the sugar bowl, and when their dad would take his first sip of coffee they would jump out and yell, "April Fool!" It was so much fun that my mother-in-law continued the joke after the girls left the nest.

If you think the use (or misuse) of seasoning isn't important, just try salt in your coffee.

Like a good trick or a joke, salt and other spices add zest to life. As far back as the book of Job, people couldn't imagine eating certain foods such as an egg without adding a little flavor:

"Is tasteless food eaten without salt, or is there flavor in the white of an egg? I refuse to touch it; such food makes me ill" (Job 6:6,7).

The Gift of Herbs and Spices

At least four Hebrew words can be translated "herb." Depending on the context in the Bible, the Hebrew words usually translated "herbs" can also be translated either grasses, sprouts, spices or vegetables.

Probably the word "plants" would best cover the diversity of herbs and spices used for seasoning. Almost every part of the plant—roots, stems, leaves, flowers, seeds, fruit—can be used as an herb or spice.

The bark and roots of many plants contain fungicides and antibacterial components that protect the plants from the adjacent soil's harmful organisms.

When dried, the medicinal parts of plants stay active for long periods of time.

Garlic is like many of the things God created for us. The more it is studied, the more amazing are the claims for its benefits.[1]

Garlic cloves are often used successfully to protect people from infections. Garlic has been shown to lower bad cholesterol and raise good cholesterol levels significantly. It is helpful in treating asthma, diabetes and high blood pressure. It stimulates the immune system, and is also a pain killer. Population studies indicate an inverse relationship between the amount of garlic consumed and the number of cancer deaths in a given population.

The more garlic you eat, the better? The research is there if you want to study it. Similar findings appear when we study many of the wonders God created for food.

Herbs and seasonings can be enjoyed fresh or dehydrated. Fresh herbs have more concentrated ingredients. You can expect to receive good nutrients from them. "Versatility" could be their middle name.

Herbs and spices are used in every culture in a variety of ways. They are an excellent way to enhance the flavors of food while cutting back on fat, salt or oils.

The more garlic is studied, the more amazing are the claims for its benefits.

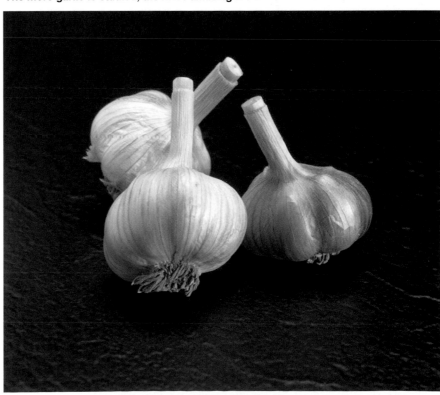

Plants, Herbs and Spices in Scripture

In the King James Version of the Bible, herbs are mentioned four times in the first chapter of Genesis. Surely they have some significance. The first two references are cited in the account of Creation:

And God said, Let the earth bring forth grass, the herb yielding seed, and the fruit tree yielding fruit after his kind, whose seed is in itself, upon the earth: and it was so. And the earth brought forth grass, and herb yielding seed after his kind, and the tree yielding fruit, whose seed was in itself, after his kind: and God saw that it was good (Gen. 1:11,12, KJV).

The fact that each plant produces after its kind indicates that these plants are similar today to the way they were when first designed. The variation we see does not represent changes in the DNA or genetic code. Variation shows the tremendous latitude the original design had.

After God created man, He said:

Behold, I have given you every

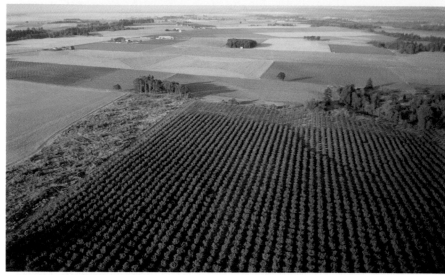

"Let the earth bring forth grass, the herb yielding seed, and the fruit tree yielding fruit."

herb bearing seed, which is upon the face of all the earth, and every tree, in the which is the fruit of a tree yielding seed; to you it shall be for meat. And to every beast of the earth, and to every fowl of the air, and to every thing that creepeth upon the earth, wherein there is life, I have given every green herb for meat: and it was so (vv. 29,30, KJV).

The Bible mentions more than 120 kinds of plants. Some of these words, such as flowers, grains and nuts, are used generically, without a specific kind being described. Other plant names, such as flax or onions, are very specific. Biblical scholars and botanists are still not 100 percent sure what plants today correlate with the biblical names.

Dr. David Darom, a botanist, has identified and photographed 80 kinds of plants mentioned in the Bible that are still growing in Israel today.[2]

"I have given you every herb bearing seed . . . and every tree, in the which is the fruit of a tree yielding seed . . ."

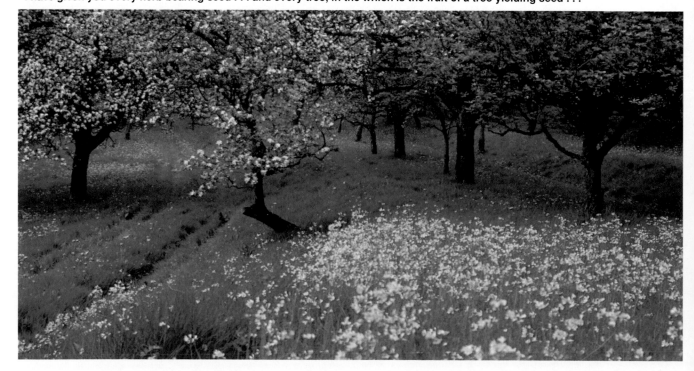

Sweet Spices as Treasure

Spices were often treasured as gifts in ancient times. When Jacob wanted to win the favor of the Egyptian Pharaoh to obtain relief from famine, he instructed his sons:

Put some of the best products of the land in your bags and take them down to the man as a gift—a little balm and a little honey, some spices and myrrh, some pistachio nuts and almonds (Gen. 43:11).

Sweet "fragrant" spices were to be used by the priests in the Old Covenant as holy oil:

"Take fragrant spices—gum resin, onycha and galbanum—and pure frankincense, all in equal amounts, and make a fragrant blend of incense, the work of a perfumer. It is to be salted and pure and sacred" (Exod. 30:34,35).

Sweet herbs and spices can be used and have little or no risk. Examples of sweet spices include gum, clover, cicely, cherry, bay, basil, alyssum, fern, flag, gale, pea, marjoram, pepper, potato, sop and william. These tasty, sweet spices can be used freely and have considerable benefits.

Caution: Bitter Herbs

Some bitter herbs are dangerous, but others are only bitter. The Passover included herbs that, although bitter, were edible:

"That same night they are to eat the meat roasted over the fire, along with bitter herbs, and bread made without yeast" (12:8).

God protected His people from the dangers of bitter herbs that are poisonous. Today, when our bitter taste buds are stimulated, caution is required. Many bitter-tasting herbs may be suitable as medicines, but even these may be toxic in uncontrolled doses.[3] Many authorities recommend professional medical advice before using bitter herbs for health purposes. Bitter herbs usually should not be taken for prolonged periods. The wild gourd *citrullus cocoynthis* has bitter fruit, and is known to be a deadly poisonous gourd, but it can be used in small doses to ease abdominal pain.[4]

A vivid example of the danger of poisonous plants occurred during the ministry of the prophet Elisha, who ordered his servants to prepare a stew for a group of prophets:

One of them went out into the fields to gather herbs and found a wild vine. He gathered some of its gourds and cut them up into the pot of stew, though no one knew what they were. The stew was poured out for the men, but as they began to eat it, they cried out, "O man of God, there is death in the pot!" And they could not eat it (2 Kings 4:39,40).

Providentially, Elisha knew an antidote for the poison. He threw flour into the pot, and the poison was rendered harmless. Isn't it nice that the gourd was bitter and the men knew to avoid the gourd soup after tasting it?

Nice design. God loves us. The sweet spices are safe, but the bitter require caution.

Spices and Stomach Problems

What about spices? Aren't they bad for ulcers, upset stomach, colitis and so on? "Bland" diets have long been prescribed by most physicians to protect the stomach from the harmful effects of spices.

Dr. Eddie Palmer, a gastroenterologist from Houston, designed an interesting study in the early 1960s.[5] I thought his experiment was a cruel joke for many of his patients. He fed ulcer patients extremely spicy foods, including hot sauce. Hot sauce and spices were inserted directly into the stomach or duodenum and placed in direct contact on the ulcers. The patients could not even feel the spices when they came in contact with the ulcer, and the ulcers healed normally. From what I know now, I suspect that the ulcers probably healed more quickly.

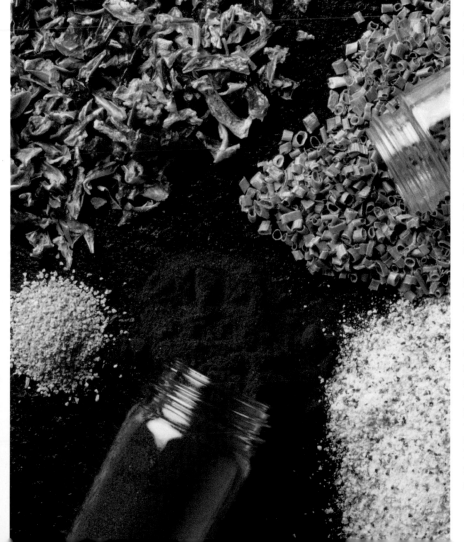

Tasty, sweet spices can be used freely and have considerable benefits.

So hot, but so healthy.

"Capsicum" is the name of a group of small shrubby plants that produce small fruits called "peppers." Cayenne is made from these dried fruits. The chemical capsaicin in pepper is what "lights our fire." It has been found to have many beneficial effects.

Capsaicin stimulates taste buds that give us a better appreciation of the food being eaten. No need for salt, sugar, fat or caffeine.

The warm sensation a person feels when eating capsaicin makes the person come back for more. The pepper fruits are loaded with essential nutrients, and many other helpful ingredients. Remember how the sweet taste attracts us to the fruits and vegetables we need. Spices may have the same attraction. They are one of the richest sources of nutrients most people eat.

In recent years, many studies on the effect of various herbs have been done. On Ovid Midline (on the Net), 95 articles in the last five years claim that hot peppers:

- Increase the metabolism so that more calories an hour are burned more efficiently;
- Relieve allergic rhinitus (runny nose);
- Act as a catalyst for other herbs;
- Improve the immune response;[6]
- Are good for healthy or diseased arteries;
- Relieve cluster headaches;
- Prevent infection;[7]
- Aid digestion;
- Help people who have asthma, emphysema and respiratory infections;
- Relieve impotence;[8]
- Warm cold feet when applied directly;
- Help relieve the pain of arthritis, pleurisy, etc.

What a Designer!

In the last 10 years since I have learned to enjoy hot stuff, I have not had one asthma attack. (I never had one the previous 40 years either.) Enjoy it hot. Enough about hot stuff.

These hot pepper claims begin to sound ridiculous; but who would believe that a little pill made of a minor ingredient found in a plant such as spiraea could relieve pain, reduce temperature, reduce inflamma-

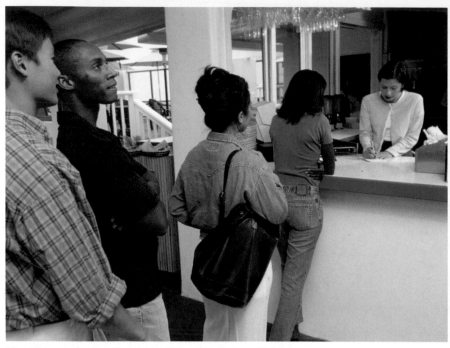

The Chinese frequently use traditional herbal medicines.

tion and reduce harmful blood clotting anywhere in the body? (Think aspirin.)

Obviously we need to remember Principle III and avoid worshiping any spice.

Spices were created not only to enhance the flavor of food and to supply nutrients, but they also have medicinal value for healing our bodies.

Eating the sprouts or young plants of wheat, alfalfa, barley[9] and other grasses has been shown to be an easy way to obtain nutrients. Like garlic, the more they are studied, the better they seem.

What About Herbal Medicine?

In all cultures, herbs are used to treat various maladies with some success. The most ancient writings of the Egyptians, Persians, Chinese and Hebrews show that herbs were used for practically every known affliction. Historically, these nations came through the Tower of Babel as grandsons of Noah.

Many of the uses of herbs were passed from one generation to the next. The Scriptures also symbolically connect herbs with healing power in the book of Revelation:

On each side of the river stood the tree of life, bearing twelve crops of fruit, yielding its fruit every month. And the leaves of the tree are for the healing of the nations (Rev. 22:2).

The prophet Jeremiah spoke of the need for spiritual healing symbolically in terms of a "balm" (an herbal treatment):

Is there no balm in Gilead? Is there no physician there? Why then is there no healing for the wound of my people? (Jer. 8:22)

Chemists have identified thousands of ingredients in herbs, many of them very powerful. The pharmaceutical industry has always isolated valuable ingredients from plants, making them available in purer forms. Today, 25 percent of all drugs still come from herbs.

Do Herbs Hint of a Design?

An apparent benefit of herbs is that they are less toxic than drugs are. Herbalists report that the drugs in herbs are buffered by other components, reducing the toxic effects while acting as a synergist. It looks like a "design" to me.

Moderation remains the key.

What is the proper balance between

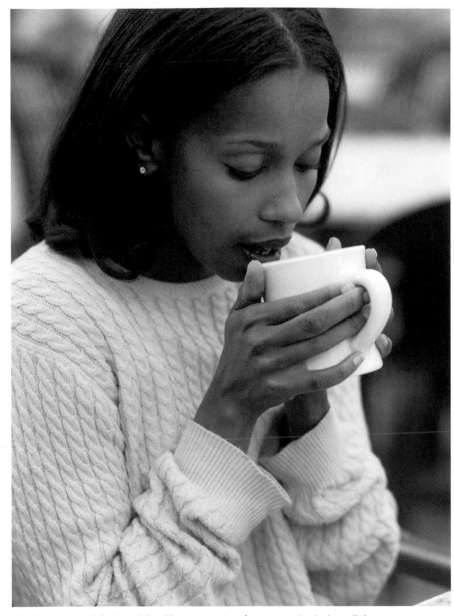

Seek your physician's advice if you are planning to use herbal medicine.

a balancing effect on these chemicals, making the herbs less toxic and improving the effectiveness of the beneficial drug they contain. Just why and how they work in this way remains something of a mystery.[10]

To ask the *why* question invites the answer that a Designer is behind this beneficial effect.

The Balm of Aloes

Some claims on behalf of the plant "aloe vera" may be hard to substantiate, but overall it does have qualities that are good for our health. Jelly from the plant seems to soothe burns, abrasions and similar problems, and to speed the healing process. Unfortunately, when chemists processed the plant to isolate its healing ingredient, the beneficial components of the plant were decreased.

Aloes are spoken of in the Bible in the good company of several prized fruits, balms and spices:

> *Your plants are an orchard of*
> *pomegranates with choice fruits,*
> *with henna and nard, nard and*
> *saffron, calamus and cinnamon,*
> *with every kind of incense tree,*
> *with myrrh and aloes and all the*
> *finest spices* (Song of Sol.
> 4:13,14).

Aloes were also a part of the blessedness God envisioned for Israel:

> *"How beautiful are your tents, O*
> *Jacob, your dwelling places, O*
> *Israel! Like valleys they spread*
> *out, like gardens beside a river,*
> *like aloes planted by the Lord, like*
> *cedars beside the waters"* (Num.
> 24:5,6).

Although I have little experience in using herbs for specific ailments, I would apply the same principles to this group of natural products that I would to the things God created for food. Because they were a part of the things God created for us, some herbs probably are a wise way to treat certain illnesses. Seek your physician's advice if you are planning to use herbs. If you don't get the desired results quickly, or if you get worse, use the best pharmaceuticals for your health problems. After a few months of following the Divine Design for health, you probably will have few times in your life when you will need to make these decisions.

herbs, physicians and pharmaceuticals?

Both traditional medicine (herbs, acupuncture, etc.) and modern medicine (pharmaceuticals, etc.) are practiced in China today. The Chinese use of herbal medicines is much more frequent than it is in the United States, but the use of pharmaceuticals is far more advanced in the United States than it is in China.

A few years ago I spoke to a group of internists and vascular surgeons in Beijing. My interpreter, a pediatrician, was well educated and involved in making medical policy for the country. Between talks I asked him how he chose between herbs and drugs in treating the sick. His response was that he and other physicians initially treat patients with herbs, and that often this relieves symptoms until the body heals itself. If the patient continues to be sick, gets worse or is critically ill, conventional pharmaceuticals are used.

Dr. James Balch, a board-certified urologist from Indiana, airs a radio program and writes a newspaper column about the subject of taking responsibility for your health. He notes that herbs have one important advantage over isolated drugs. Herbs contain powerful chemicals that treat specific health problems. Yet they also have many other ingredients that have

The Savor of Salt

Salt is the *numero uno* seasoning in the world. Jesus' reference to it in the Sermon on the Mount has also most likely made salt the best-known food product mentioned in Scripture. Although Jesus spoke approvingly of salt, He added something that reminds us of Principle II:

"You are the salt of the earth. But if the salt loses its saltiness, how can it be made salty again? It is no longer good for anything, except to be thrown out and trampled by men" (Matt. 5:13).

There are two main sources of salt: rock salt and powder salt (including sea salt). Rock salt is taken from thick layers of sedimentary rock. This sediment was probably formed by a worldwide flood. (Have you ever heard of such a catastrophic event?) All of the mined salt appears to be sodium chloride (NaCl). Several varieties are sold, including table salt, rock salt and kosher salt.

In the United States, 70 percent of salt consumption comes from salt being added to food by food handlers. Therefore, it goes without too much analysis that we eat too much salt.

It is easy to become addicted to salt. Enough evidence of possible health risks exist to make it advisable for most people to cut back on their use of salt.

What About Sea Salt?

The second source, sea salt, is recovered from salt water. Most commercial sea salt comes from France; sea salt is a good product. Research has proved that sea water contains many important minerals such as calcium, magnesium, potassium and manganese. The concentration of these elements in sea water is in similar proportions to that found in the human body. Sea salt is therefore perfectly designed for our use.

On the other hand, most other salt contains only sodium and chloride. Although these elements have been implicated in hypertension, recent research shows that the condition improves when patients supplement their diet with calcium, magnesium or potassium—the additional elements found in sea water. These elements are also found in vegetables and other foods. Salt would probably be of little consequence if we were receiving the minerals from foods as God designed them, or from sea water.

Unfortunately, some sea salt has been processed to near uselessness. Some brands I have tested in our lab contained only sodium and chloride; magnesium was added as an anticaking agent, but no other minerals were added.

Most brands of "sea salt" contain only sodium chloride (NaCl). A few brands retain all of the nutrients—for example, DeSouza's Salt of the Earth, and the Sea, vegetable salt mixes, and seaweed and salt mixes. My current recommendation is to use sea salt by using the same precautions you would with regular salt. Again, moderation is the key.

A wide range of synthetic flavors have been developed to mimic not only salt, but natural spices as well, particularly those of fruits. The most widely used imitation spice flavor is synthetic vanillin, which is made with flavoring agents derived from the hydrolysis of wood alcohol. Why not use real vanilla?

Most of humans' substitutes for the spices and herbs God designed are petroleum by-products, and have the same disadvantages of the other "naked" processed products such as sugar, lipids (oil) and salt. Avoid them.

12. Beverages: Elixirs of Life— or Death

Life's elixir—water—is the basis of beverages, and a God-designed essential of all life.

An inquisitive four-year-old girl was "helping" her mother prepare a meal for several guests one evening. She reached up to the stove to shake a skillet filled with searing-hot grease. The skillet tipped, spilling scalding grease on the little girl. She screamed, her chest and abdomen covered with hot grease. Severe burns were developing, but over the girl's vigorous protest, ice and water were immediately applied. Within a few minutes the developing burns were arrested. Soon she was playing again. She suffered no blisters, no loss of skin; no skin grafts, no visits to the burn wards were needed and no scars remained.

What Is It with Water?

Play detective. Pick the property of water that prevented the little girl's burns. What quality in water could reverse her injury so fast?

It would seem that water is so "attuned" to the needs of the little girl's skin that the two substances were immediately compatible. That's exactly the case. People are composed of 65 percent water. Compare this with an ear of corn or an elephant— which are composed of 70 percent water. A tomato contains 95 percent water.

Beverages are all primarily composed of water. A small quantity of chemistry and content make the difference between milk and, say, fruit juice. Both are mostly water.

Humans can live one or two months without food, but only a few days without water.

Water is a combination of two gases bonded together by electrons. Water is the most common substance on earth. For all practical purposes, water is found on no other planet, nor on any star in the universe. One of the best evidences that life is not present on other planets is the absence of water.

Beverages are simply solids or gases dissolved in water. These solids or gases may be nutrients that are essential for life and healthy bacteria. The beverage or water, however, may contain harmful waste, toxins, germs, chemicals or mud. In 1994, 53 million Americans drank polluted water, resulting in 400,000 illnesses;[1] but clean water's unique properties are necessary for all forms of life.

No other substance can do all the things H_2O can do; it is an exception to many of nature's rules.

Water is found in all three of its physical forms—ice, liquid and gas— at temperatures normally found in the earth's atmosphere.

All chemical compounds similar to H_2O, such as hydrogen sulfide (H_2S), hydrogen telluride (H_2Te) and hydrogen selenide (H_2Se), are gases until the temperature reaches $-140°F$—then they become liquid. This unique capacity of water to become a liquid at higher temperatures is vital.

Water and God's Design

Let your mind wander a few minutes with me. What if earth were twice as far from the sun as it is now? There would be no life on earth, just ice.

What if earth were as close to the sun as is Mars, Venus or Mercury? Life would not exist on earth—just steam.

Earth is placed exactly the distance from the sun where it must be to have the necessary temperature for water to perform as a life-giving force. Is it luck or Design that we are located in space right where we are, in precisely the place where life can exist?

Ice has many unique qualities; but the one that seems to go against natural law is that it expands instead of shrinks when it changes from liquid to solid. This causes ice to float. If ice did not expand as all other molecules do during their transitions from liquid to solid, it would sink. The earth would soon be a lifeless, frozen tundra. All bodies of water would freeze from the bottom up, destroying all life in the water.

Thank You, Lord, for this one exception to the norm found in the water You so carefully designed.

Dissolvability

Another property of water that is most important to our discussion of beverages is its dissolving ability. Water can dissolve almost anything, including rock. Water dissolves nutrients and food so they are distributed to the cells in our bodies.

Heat Capacity

Back to the little girl and the scalding grease. Any clues yet to the mystery of the water cure? The answer lies in the heat capacity of water.

Heat capacity is the ability of a substance to absorb heat without elevating its temperature. Water is a champ at heat capacity (along with ammonia). If all heat were removed from a pound of iron and a pound of water by lowering the temperature to

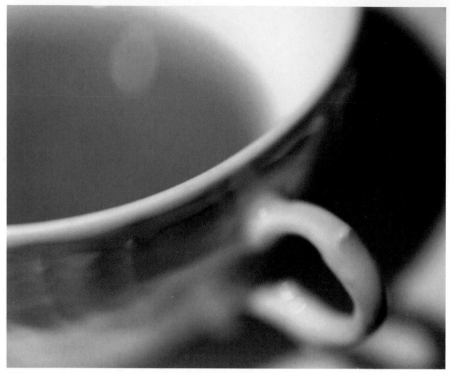

Juices and decaffeinated herbal teas added to water are good thirst quenchers.

we should drink is concerned. Dew is the equivalent to distilled water. A reverse osmosis filter also gives water that would compare to the dew from heaven. Spring water, well water and bottled water may also be fine.

Adding a touch of honey, lemon or lime to water can be pleasant to the taste buds. Various juices and decaffeinated herbal teas added to water are good thirst quenchers. Honey-lemonade and freshly squeezed fruit juices provide exceptionally good products for drinking.

Drinking pure water or water that contains natural flavorings certainly adheres to Principle I.

What About Chlorinated Water?

The Bible also says:
So Israel will live in safety alone; Jacob's spring is secure in a land of grain and new wine, where the heavens drop dew (v. 28).

Having a "secure spring" is a necessity for prolonged healthy living. We need clean, pure water. Yet contaminated water supplies are not unusual. Water's dissolving ability makes us vulnerable to all kinds of contamination. Remember the women dying after childbirth in Austria (beginning of chapter 1)? It wasn't the young mothers' fault that their caregivers were ignorant of God's commands. Precautions could have been taken. We need to be careful that the H_2O we drink is pure.

Tests show that many cities have water purity problems. According to the *Los Angeles Times*, this is enough of a problem in Los Angeles that a survey of the Los Angeles City Water Department discovered 59 percent of its employees drink bottled or filtered water.

Environmental Protection Agency studies show high levels of contamination in Charleston, South Carolina; Houston, Texas; Oklahoma City, Oklahoma; Tampa, Florida; and many other communities in our country.[2]

–273°F.; then if equal amounts of heat were applied to each, the iron would reach 2,370°—its melting point; at the same time water would reach 32°—its melting point. The point is that water has a greater capacity than iron to absorb heat.

Geographically, this means that the earth, whose surface is more than 70 percent water, will have little variation in temperature between night and day, especially in areas where water is prevalent.

As far as humans are concerned, this also means that our bodies—which contain 65 percent water—have stable temperatures. A swing of as little as 8° in the body's temperature can be fatal.

This is the big clue to why water helped the inquisitive young girl. The 65 percent water content of her skin absorbed a lot of the calories from the hot oil before permanent damage was done to her skin's enzymes and cells. The ice water thrown on the skin also had tremendous capacity to draw the heat from the hot oil and the hot skin.

Conclusion: Apply ice-cold water on any burn as quickly as possible. You have little time before severe damage is done.

Beverages and The Three Principles

Let's take a brief survey of beverages mentioned in the Bible, keeping The Three Principles in mind:

Principle I: Eat only substances God created for food.

Principle II: As much as possible, eat foods as they were created—before they are changed or converted into something humans think might be better.

Principle III: Avoid food addictions. Don't let any food or drink become your god.

The Treasure of Pure Water

In Deuteronomy 33, God promised that His people would live,
in a land of grain and new wine, where the heavens drop dew (v. 28).

Dew is pure water. That is the key message for us today as far as what

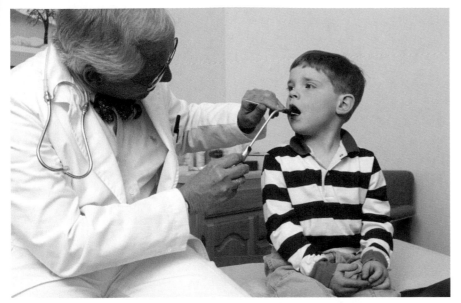

Many toothpastes warn against using too much because of possible fluoride toxicity.

So it is a good idea to check your water. Remember:

Prove all things; hold fast that which is good (1 Thess. 5:21, KJV).

Most water suppliers have made great efforts to prevent bacterial contamination. The primary method involves water chlorination. Chlorine kills bacteria and does it well. Unfortunately, it is toxic to our cells as well. Chlorine poses many theoretical dangers to humans. One book that will scare you is titled *Coronaries/Cholesterol/Chlorine* by Joseph M Price, M.D.[3] Dr. Price, who is a biochemist, shows that adding chlorine to water is an example of violating Principle II. Yet it is not hard to avoid chlorine. Simple filtering, stirring or letting the water sit for a few hours will allow this gas to escape from the water.

The Debate About Fluoride

The use of fluoride is an explosive, emotional, debatable, controversial and difficult issue. Do you get the idea that I have friends and family who are stalwarts on both sides of this issue?

The American Dental Association and the American Medical Association support the research that claims fluoride prevents cavities.[4] Most cities add

it to their water supplies. It is added to toothpaste, and to anything that contains water. Most of our processed foods therefore contain fluoride.

No one denies that fluoride can be toxic at certain levels. The president of the American Pediatric Dental Association recommended in 1992 that parents not put more than one little drop of fluoride toothpaste on a child's toothbrush because of the product's potential toxicity.[5] Most toothpaste containers warn against using too much toothpaste because of possible fluoride toxicity.

Plenty of children who ingest fluoride water still get cavities. Our son had cavities every visit he made to the dentist during his first six years. His toothpaste contained fluoride and it was also present in the water he drank. No matter how many times a day his mother brushed and flossed his teeth, the cavities just kept on coming. His grandfather—a dentist—tried every old and new idea to prevent the cavities. This wasn't just an ordinary problem—the cavities became abscesses that required antibiotic treatment.

From the time we started eating whole foods and avoided naked calories, one of the unexpected bonuses was that our son had no more cavities for at least 12 years. His younger brother also benefited to the same degree. My conclusion is that cavities are caused primarily by "naked calories."

Once again, in my experience, if we eat the things created for food before they are changed into nutrient-deficient naked calories, we will reap great benefits.

The Beverage That Is a Food

Then we have the universal beverage-food—milk.

In Genesis 18:8, Abraham hosted three men (or angels) representing God Himself. The Bible says:

[Abraham] took butter, and milk, and the calf which he had dressed, and set it before them; and he stood by them under the tree, and they did eat (KJV).

In Deuteronomy 32:14, God brought to Jacob,

Butter of kine, and milk of sheep, with fat of lambs, and rams of the breed of Bashan, and goats, with the fat of kidneys of wheat (KJV).

Although clean milk is another excellent beverage given to us by the Creator, health advisors frequently offer opposing advice. The American Dairy Association says we need several glasses of milk every day. Others say that no milk should be consumed past infancy. In between is the skim-milk, no-fat gang.

Still others say we should consume goat's milk only. God has provided this beverage, too:

And thou shalt have goats' milk enough for thy food, for the food of thy household, and for the maintenance for thy maidens (Prov. 27:27, KJV).

Let's take a closer look at milk—its benefits for both infants and adults.

What About Nursing?

Psalm 8:2 states:

Out of the mouth of babes and sucklings hast thou ordained strength (KJV).

It is assumed in the Bible that breast milk is good for babies; however, about 40 to 50 years ago some scientists decided that human milk was deficient in both Vitamin D and iron. Various formulas containing supplemental iron and Vitamin D were recommended, and most infants during those years received these formulas instead of nursing their mothers.

That thinking has since been challenged. In a recent article about breast feeding, Dr. Paul Palma discussed the increased bioavailability of several micronutrients (iron, vitamin D, zinc, etc.) when presented to the infant's digestive system in the exact balance found in human breast milk.[6] These micronutrients are utilized by the infant much more efficiently than with any possible supplementation.

If the human milk is pasteurized, much of the bioavailability is lost. Could this happen in other kinds of milk also? Palma also noted that breast milk has a perfect nutrient balance of macronutrients (lipids, protein, carbohydrates), which change as the needs of a premature, mature or growing infant's needs change.

Infants who have been breast-fed have been studied up to five years of age. They have a much lower incidence of diarrhea, urinary tract infections, pneumonia, vomiting, asthma, earaches, childhood allergies and crib death. Also, viral and bacterial infections, cancers and learning disabilities are less of a problem. Parents of these children may be spared much anguish and also avoid costly medical care.

In one study, the incidence of breast cancer was shown to be decreased by 25 percent in women proportional to the amount of time they have breast-fed infants during their lives.[7]

Psychological, mental and immunological benefits have also been documented. Breast feeding entails close contact with tactile, auditory, olfactory and visual interchange, all of which reinforce the maternal-infant bonding. This bonding between mother and infant may be more important than the other advantages of breast milk.

The longer the duration of breast feeding, the more measurable the improvement in the quality of the mother-child relationship for as long as two years after birth. A lowered risk of syndromes such as child abuse or failure to thrive also are benefits. The father's support is also invaluable in fostering successful bonding.

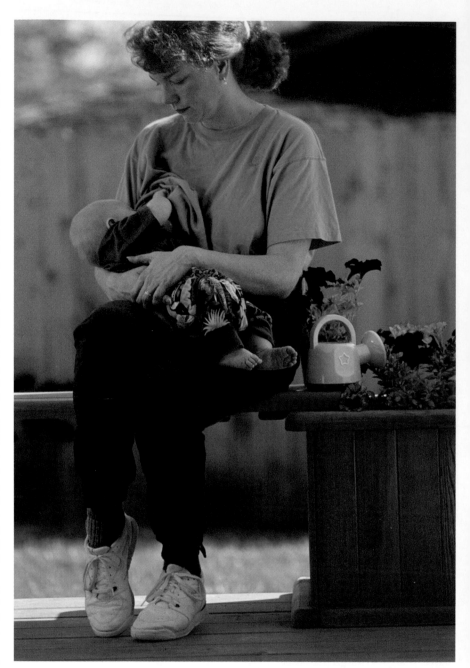

Human milk is truly living fluid in which antibodies and cells move.

Our reasons for using formulas appeared to be correct and more convenient. Formula-fed children, however, lost the protection and strength of human breast milk. In other words, choosing a human's way rather than God's design proved to be poor judgment. How many have suffered because humans thought they had better ideas and recommended formulas containing supplements instead of the real thing? The value of a formula today is measured by how close it can compare to the mother's milk. Formulas really do not compare to breast milk.

Nursing and God's Design

Most scientists claim that life came from a random chance process and by natural selection. In nature, however, a chorus of voices ring with the message that this theory fits neither simple nor complex observations. To maintain health, the following must be present simultaneously and in proper balance: organic vitamins, minerals, essential fatty acids, essential amino acids and unrefined carbohydrates. These are all present in human breast milk, as are hundreds harmful to the baby, but apparently they have the ability to produce antibodies that destroy bacteria and viruses as well. Apparently the infant who is exposed to infections, then nurses from its mother, produces changes in the mother's breast. Within hours, the next milk starts producing antibodies and immunoglobulins to protect the baby before the infant becomes sick.

Where would the human race be if the first baby had no mother's breast to suck? What if just one of several specific enzymes to allow digestion of the lactose, lipids or proteins found in her milk were missing? What if one of the essential amino acids, fatty acids, vitamins, minerals, etc., were not in a bioavailable form or in optimal concentrations in the first mother's milk? Humankind would not have existed through one generation. Certainly a Designer is a necessity. Random chance equals no chance. The time (eons) for developing the essentials for life in milk would equal death for any species. We need the complete product from the beginning.

What About Pasteurization?

Would you believe that the sale of pasteurized milk was against the law for years because it was associated with health problems? The process of pasteurization involves heating a liquid to 160° for 45 minutes. Originally, the technique was used for wine, but eventually dairies discovered how it could help them.

Did scientific discovery change the law? No, political lobbying did. Read *The Milk of Human Kindness Is Not Pasteurized* by William Campbell Douglass, M.D.[8] Dr. Douglass's book documents one of the best examples of Principle II: eat foods as they were created—before they are changed or converted into something humans think might be better.

Dr. Douglass agrees with our principle, insisting that we should drink milk prior to processing, which changes it into a nutrient-deficient product.

Before it is pasteurized, whole milk

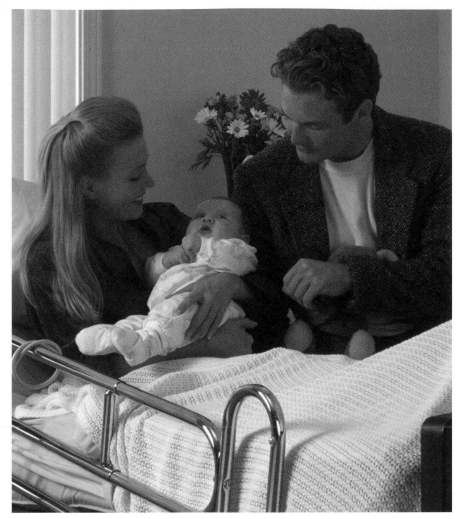

Breast-fed children have a special resistance to many childhood diseases.

of other lesser understood food factors. The longer scientists study the human breast and its milk, the more obvious it is that neither random chance nor survival of the fittest could explain its complexity.

The design of the milk is perfect in caloric content, amino acid concentrations and enzyme concentrations. Both lipase and lactase are ideally concentrated, meeting the developing infant's needs much better than could any formula or other mammal's milk.

The caloric content and the nutrient balance of the mother's milk change dramatically according to the infant's needs. Our most brilliant neonatologists using the best computers could not design a better balanced product than breast milk, regardless of the infant's needs at whatever age or stage of development.

The case of premature infants is instructive. It is now known that during the first month of lactation the nitrogen and protein content declines in most mothers' milk content. The milk of a mother who gave birth to a premature infant, however, is as much as 20 percent higher in proteins. It seems this weak, premature baby would be culled out by the law of survival of the fittest. Instead, a loving God designed special milk to meet the premature infant's needs.

Survival of the fittest? Why would a random process protect the weak, premature infant with such a intricately designed changing milk?

Breast-fed children have a special resistance to many childhood diseases. This is because the early milk or colostrum sets up the infant's immunoreactive system. The early milk contains two classes of immunoactive components: cells and soluble protein factors. Human milk is truly living fluid in which antibodies and cells move. The cells in the mother's milk not only attack bacteria that may be contains many healthy proteins, enzymes, vitamins and minerals. A prime example is the vitamin folic acid. A 1982 study reported that pasteurization denatures enzymes, decreasing the bioavailability of the folic acid and other nutrients found in raw milk.[9] The heating in the process also destroys some of the vitamins and nutrients. The altered protein probably results in some people being allergic to dairy products. Calcium absorption is also decreased.

To suggest drinking unpasteurized milk scares some people tremendously. The reason for pasteurization is to kill bacteria, and what we need is clean milk from a healthy cow rather than pasteurization. Clean milk can be produced and transported in a healthful manner today. Certainly the incidents of brucellosis or tuberculosis being transmitted in milk is very low.

In 1920, when pasteurization was first implemented, 65 percent of all cows had tuberculosis and 15 percent had brucellosis.

According to a phone conversation with Jack Mathis, president of Mathis Dairy in Decatur, Georgia, recently, the Centers for Disease Control in Atlanta collected 18 cases of brucellosis across the United States in one year. In each of those cases, the infection occurred because of contamination of the patient's blood or mucous membranes from the cow's feces. This mainly happened to veterinarians, but also to some cattle handlers who had been contaminated with fecal material as they worked with the animals.

Although the number of persons already drinking raw milk (without homogenization or pasteurization) cannot be determined, it is known that many dairy farmers and their families do drink raw milk. There are 11 million dairy cows in the United States. If only a small percentage of these families use their own cows' milk, the number of persons drinking raw milk probably numbers in the thousands. The Mathis dairy in Atlanta, Georgia, sells huge amounts of clean raw milk that is carefully scrutinized by the FDA. No cases of brucellosis or other contamination are being transmitted by drinking this milk. The health risk remains low if clean milk is produced.

Every few years a local outbreak of

Getting the Most from Milk

	Pasteurized	Raw
Vitamin C	50% lost	All present
Enzymes	10% remain	All present
Amino acids	Lysine and tyrosine altered	All 22 AAs present
Fatty acids	Fatty acids altered	All FAs retained
Vitamins A and D	2/3 lost	Unaltered
Vitamin B-complex	40-80% lost	Unaltered
Minerals: Calcium and magnesium	50% lost	100% bioavailable*

*Note: Calcium and magnesium require enzymes present in raw milk for best absorption.

listeria or salmonella infections occur when milk consumption is a primary factor. Most cases I have seen reported, however, were caused from drinking pasteurized milk. Pasteurization does not guarantee that the milk will be clean.[10] The FDA only requires a bacteria count of less than 75,000 per cubic centimeter of Grade A milk. By heating, or pasteurizing, the count is dropped to about 25,000; but the count may be back up by the time it is sold—and it will still be considered Grade A milk. You may get sick when harmful bacteria are present.

Certified raw milk, on the other hand, has to contain bacteria counts of less than 10,000—and raw milk can earn this certification easily if it is clean. Yet that dairy in Atlanta is one of the few certified dairies in the United States from which raw milk may be legally sold. You people in Georgia should enjoy it.

This certified dairy is inspected daily, which is much more frequent than inspections of conventional dairy operations. The requirements in producing this uncontaminated milk mean that the work areas must meet stringent cleanliness standards—almost as strict as a surgical suite in a hospital—and the cows must be maintained in excellent health.

A study by Dr. E. V. McCollum, a biochemist from Johns Hopkins University, revealed many interesting facts, some of which are summarized in the chart above.[11]

The decision about whether to drink only raw but certified milk is one that has to be made individually. Because of current governmental restraints about the use of raw milk, it is not available to most of us.

So why do I bother to tell you these things? Because we often pray in desperation: Why me Lord? Why my loved one? "My people are destroyed [die needlessly] from lack of knowledge" (Hos. 4:6). Clean cow's milk and clean goat's milk are some of the most complete health-giving foods on earth.

What About Homogenization?

Proverbs 30:33 says:
Surely the churning of milk bringeth forth butter, and the wringing of the nose bringeth forth blood (KJV).

I use this verse to respond to critics who say the Bible is not true. Just offer to twist their noses to see if blood comes forth. It will! This is another biblical truth illustrated.

The point here, though, is that by biblical definition homogenized dairy products may no longer be milk, because churning homogenized milk won't bring forth butter.

Homogenization breaks up the larger butterfat globules in whole

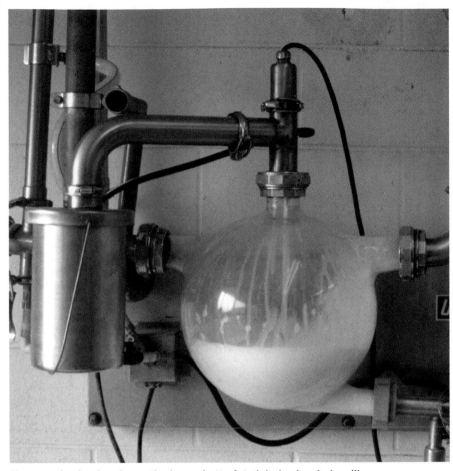

Homogenization breaks up the larger butterfat globules in whole milk.

milk into very tiny globules, which suspends them evenly in the milk. This means the milk doesn't require stirring when it is stored, and may add to the storage life of the product. The resulting modification, however, may point to one of the contributing factors for the large increase in vascular disease in the United States.

The normal larger butterfat molecules in nonhomogenized milk bounce through the intestine, and only small portions are absorbed as they travel through the intestines because of the limited surface area in contact with the mucosa of the small bowel. The smaller particles of butterfat resulting from homogenization create a marked increase in the surface area of butterfat presented to the mucosa of the small bowel. The small particles pass quickly into the bloodstream. The result is that nearly all of the fat in homogenized milk enters the bloodstream, raising our triglycerides and cholesterol levels unnecessarily, according to Jack Mathis.

According to Dr. Kurt A. Oster of Yale University, an important enzyme in butterfat (xanthine oxidase) is capable of digesting the intima layer of arteries (lining), causing ulcers inside our arteries.[12]

On the other hand, small ulcers in the intima are healed by cholesterol, causing a small plaque. This plaque causes swelling and thickening of the intima. Eventually calcium is added to the cholesterol deposits. This progression can cause strictures that may block the vessels or cause thrombosis. A small plaque may detach at any time, causing sudden blockage of the artery.

During the Vietnam War in Southeast Asia, autopsies of young American soldiers revealed a high incidence of ulcers in the intima of their vessels, and even more advanced plaques in their arteries. The same age Vietnamese soldiers had no disease in their arteries. These findings, along with other population studies around the world, implicate homogenized milk.

Recently in Japan the comparative effects of milk, yogurt, butter and margarine on breast tumors was studied.[13] It was discovered that butter protected from breast tumors, while margarine enhanced the development of breast tumors. Because butter comes from milk, we might assume that milk and yogurt would also be beneficial. To the researchers' surprise, the opposite was true. Why? Could it be that pasteurizing or homogenizing milk caused this change in expected benefit? More tests are being designed. I predict that raw milk, like butter, will prevent breast tumors, while the processed milk will do the opposite.

Milk Products and Substitutes

Pure butter, kefir and their products, such as homemade ice cream and cheeses, are God-given, healthful products. Commercial skim milk can be used in cooking.

Yogurts are generally healthful products, unless producers add a lot of sugar to them. It is generally better to buy plain yogurt and mix in whatever fruits you prefer.

Principles II and III cause me to avoid homogenized and pasteurized milk products, particularly commercially processed cheeses, ice creams, milk sherbets and instant breakfasts. Processed cheeses usually contain many added chemicals, and ice creams may be similarly modified.

What About Alcoholic Beverages?

The Christian community has long been divided about the issue of alcoholic beverages. There are many reasons for this: (a) Christians come from many different social cultures—some condone and some condemn drinking alcoholic beverages; (b) there are enormous personal and social costs of alcohol abuse, because alcohol is such an addictive substance; (c) the Bible does not provide an absolute prohibition against any alcohol use, although it does provide ample and repeated warnings about the abuse of wine and strong drink.

As we have seen, the Bible mentions several kinds of drink: water, milk, juice, wine and strong drink. Obviously, there is no controversy about water or milk. The word "juice" (*asis*) is barely controversial, because it is used only once to describe making spiced wine from the juice of pomegranates (see Song of Sol. 8:2).

There is also little controversy that *sekar*, "strong drink," means a fermented intoxicating beverage. In all but one case (see Num. 28:7; compare with Num. 28:14 and Exod. 29:40), *sekar* is a strong drink other than wine (see examples in Lev. 10:9; Num. 6:3; Deut. 14:26; Prov. 20:1; Isa. 24:9). Whether *sekar* was beer or something stronger, it was capable of making someone drunk (see Gen. 9:21; Isa. 29:9; Jer. 25:27).

The controversy revolves around the words translated into English as "wine." The two words most commonly used for wine in the Old Testament are *yayin* (used 141 times), and *tirosh* (used 38 times). *Yayin* is usually translated "wine" and *tirosh* is often translated "new wine." Some biblical commentaries suggest that *yayin* is wine fermented from the previous year, and *tirosh* is a somewhat less fermented drink from the recent harvest.

Others concede that *yayin* is a fermented and intoxicating beverage, but *tirosh* is simply freshly squeezed juice from grapes.[14] The exact nature of "wine" and "new wine" is not absolutely clear in the Old Testament. From Hosea 4:11, however, we know that along with harlotry, both *yayin* and *tirosh* are capable of taking away understanding. The disciples in Acts 2:13 (KJV) were accused of being drunk with "new wine." It is possible that some of the time *tirosh* may not have had alcoholic content, and could have been similar to freshly squeezed grape juice.

Both *yayin* and *tirosh* are blessings from God that gladden a person's heart (*yayin*: see Ps. 104:15; Judg. 9:13; Eccles. 2:3, 9:7, 10:19; Zech. 9:17; 10:7; and *tirosh*: see Gen.

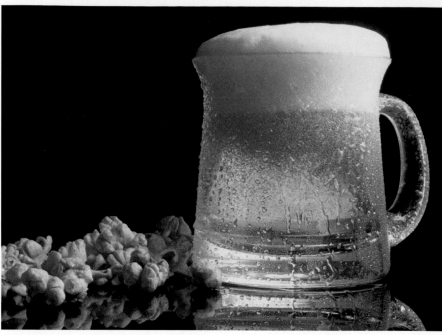

The Bible gives repeated warnings about the abuse of strong drink.

27:28; Deut. 7:13; 33:28). Significant restrictions, however, were placed on the use of wine: priests could not drink while doing their priestly duties (see Lev. 10:9); Nazirites took vows never to drink wine or the fruit of the vine (see Num. 6:3; cf. Judg. 13:4,7,14); leaders were wise to avoid addiction to wine (see Prov. 20:1; 21:17; 31:4).

For example,
Who has woe? Who has sorrow? Who has strife? Who has complaints? Who has needless bruises? Who has bloodshot eyes? Those who linger over wine, who go to sample bowls of mixed wine. Do not gaze at wine when it is red, when it sparkles in the cup, when it goes down smoothly! In the end it bites like a snake and poisons like a viper (Prov. 23:29-32).
The Old Testament admonishes against becoming drunk, whether drunkenness is caused by strong drink or by wine (e.g., see Isa. 5:11; Hab. 2:5; 1 Sam. 1:15).

The most common New Testament word for wine is *oinos*. On the one hand, wine is a gift to be enjoyed, as we see from Jesus' first public miracle (see John 2:1-11). Jesus was even accused by His enemies of being "a glutton and a drunkard" (Matt. 11:18,19). In the New Testament, however, drunkenness is a character-

istic of Gentiles who do not know God (see 1 Pet. 4:3). Rather than be drunk with wine, Christians are to be filled with the Holy Spirit (see Eph. 5:18). For the sake of the progress of the gospel, it may be necessary to refrain from drinking wine (see Rom. 14:21). Wine was recognized as having medicinal value (see 1 Tim. 5:23; see also 2 Sam. 16:1,2; Luke 10:34; Mark 15:23), but it was imperative that church leaders not be overdependent on wine (see 1 Tim. 3:1-3,8).

Modern Cautions About Enjoyment of "New Wine"

New wine or fresh juices are a gift from God to be enjoyed. The only caution would be to monitor the volume consumed, particularly if someone has a tendency toward diabetes. The sugar content of one glass of juice equals three apples.

The high potassium content in fruit juice is also beneficial for high blood pressure and for the cardiac muscle. Those who have high potassium content in their tissues show more resistance to cancer, and those who have cancer often have low potassium levels. Eating fresh vegetables or fruit will help raise the potassium level. Bananas are one of the best sources of natural potassium.

In Bible times, good wines were

valued highly and were usually diluted to a ratio of one part wine to three or four parts water.[15] I recommend a similar practice.

What About Fermented Wine?

Many juices turn to wine while being stored. Some juices turn to wine if yeast is added. Some authorities say the alcohol content of wines in Bible times was usually around 1 percent, a percentage of alcohol that inhibits contamination by bacteria. In New Testament times, wine was often safer to drink than water was.

I am not naive enough to think that early humans did not know how to increase the alcohol content. Certainly the stuff Noah drank was not diluted four parts to one. Today, because large amounts of sugar are added to wines, the alcohol content is much higher, some wines containing 10 to 20 percent alcohol.

For those who enjoy the taste of wine but want to avoid alcohol, de-alcoholized wine is available. Like alcoholic wine, it increases the absorption of potassium, calcium, magnesium, phosphorous and zinc. Freshly squeezed fruit juices also cause the same absorbing benefits. The alcohol in other wines promotes the excretion of these same minerals that really need to be absorbed—further indicating that de-alcoholized wines or fresh fruit juices are better than fermented wine and other alcoholic drinks.

Health Benefits and Liabilities of Wines

Freshly squeezed fruit juices and fermented wine contain about 200 other substances that I believe are beneficial to our digestion and nutrition. Although many of these associated food factors are not completely understood yet, we do know that juices and wines contain simple and complex carbohydrates, minerals, vitamins, amino acids and enzymes. Both fresh and fermented wines have beneficial ingredients such as antiviral agents. This antiviral effect may lie behind the well-known New Testament passage in which Paul counsels the younger minister Timothy about wine being beneficial for soothing an upset stomach (see

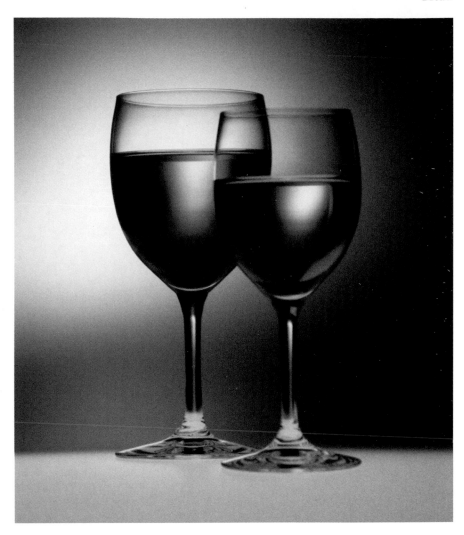

Alcohol is a depressant of the central nervous system.

1 Tim. 5:23).

Today, however, it should be added that alcoholic wine raises the blood pressure, in addition to causing many other problems.

Alcohol is a depressant of the central nervous system. It suppresses the immune system. It blocks proper nutrient absorption. It alters enzymes that normally protect us from cancer. It causes birth defects. It depletes B vitamins as well as substantial amounts of minerals. It impedes glycogen (fitness fuel) storage in the liver. Athletes are stupid to imbibe because alcohol impairs coordination and reduces the contraction of muscles.

This list can go on almost indefinitely. It gets boring.

As an eighth-grade student, I remember writing a book report about *Alcohol the Destroyer.* After studying that book, I wondered why, if we know all detrimental effects, do people

and the government allow the continued consumption of alcohol?

During all of my years of study since that book report, only a few reports have shown any good effects of alcohol. In 1994, the University of Wisconsin reinforced the idea that red wine may help prevent heart attacks. Actually, the beneficial ingredients are the flavinoids, which are found in higher concentrations in the skins, stems and seed of grapes, as well as in other fruits, vegetables and tea. These compounds reduce abnormal blood clotting, which may cause heart attacks and strokes, but they have higher concentrations in juice, fruits and some vegetables than they do in wine.

The wine industry is clever. Every three or four years a news release reports part of the story about the protective effects of their product. These releases usually come after reports that the sale of wine is decreasing again.

The only thing unhealthy about wine is its alcohol content. Alcohol is a two-carbon carbohydrate that is dangerous. Literally thousands of research articles document the ill effects of this compound. Researchers at the University of Chicago found that within an hour after a few drinks, the heart's performance will be depressed. In their experiments, the muscle fiber of the left ventricle did not perform as well as it did before the men drank alcohol.

At Thomas Jefferson University, similar studies show that consumption of alcohol leads to a number of harmful alterations in the contractile function of the heart's muscle.[16]

In another study, ethyl alcohol decreased flow through the coronary arteries and produced angina and electrocardiographic (ECG) changes in patients that have stable angina.[17]

Medical Warnings Against "Strong Drink"

"Strong drink" can do serious damage to the human body. If a pregnant woman drinks even a little alcohol during pregnancy, it passes through the mother and into the fetus growing within the mother, producing birth defects or fetal alcohol syndrome. This condition, called "FAS," produces newborn babies that have mental and physical retardation, deformed heads and faces, heart diseases and/or spinal cord and brain malformations.

Some health reports indicate that alcohol may lower cholesterol slightly. Big deal! Contrast that slight benefit with the multiple hazards produced when alcohol "burns" into the heart muscle of thousands of newborn infants. Women who consume alcohol during an extended time period definitely increase the risk of heart failure in their children.

Recently a team led by a Harvard researcher discovered three amazing proteins in embryos that control the left-hand/right-hand patterning.[18] One kind of protein completely different from the other is found on the left-hand side of the body. All nutrients coming into the embryo through this protein are used to build the left side of the body. Another protein builds the right arm. Other precise proteins

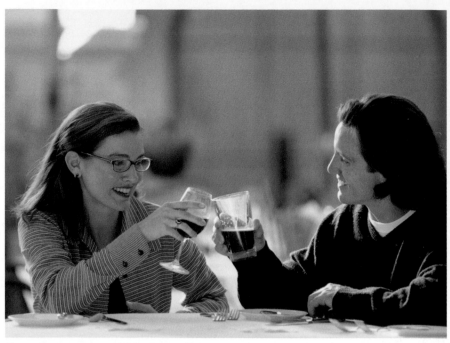

If a pregnant woman drinks even a little alcohol, it passes into the fetus, producing possible birth defects.

direct chemicals to build the elbow between the upper arm and forearm.

Do you remember how complex the formation of one single protein is? If one amino acid gets out of place, that structural change can destroy the developing organs or extremity. Alcohol denatures protein on contact. It is amazing that any baby can develop normally; why add to the risk by ingesting anything that adds to the risk?

Alcohol causes damage to the human brain, joints, muscles and to every organ system in the body. Why not avoid alcohol, especially because the Creator warns us. Is there any reason to use alcohol? According to Scripture, there is at least one use for it:

Give beer [strong drink] to those who are perishing, wine to those who are in anguish; let them drink and forget their poverty and remember their misery no more (Prov. 31:6,7).

But if our aim in life is not to fall into poverty or to deliberately perish, alcohol is a great substance to avoid. We must take to heart the reference to the human body as a "temple," as Paul said:

Do you not know that your body is a temple of the Holy Spirit, who is in you, whom you have received from God? (1 Cor. 6:19).

Alcoholic wine also contains sulfites—antifoaming agents, copper sulfate, ferrocyanide compounds and propylene glycol, all of which cause damage to our health. These are just a bunch of chemicals that have been added for various reasons.

Does it make sense to pour this liquid, which has many hazards warned against in both scientific and scriptural sources, into our "temples"?

Perhaps the most serious danger of alcohol is its mental and addictive effects, which Proverbs also describes very well:

In the end it bites like a snake and poisons like a viper. Your eyes will see strange sights and your mind imagine confusing things. You will be like one sleeping on the high seas, lying on top of the rigging. "They hit me," you will say, "but I'm not hurt! They beat me, but I don't feel it! When will I wake up so I can find another drink?" (Prov. 23:32-35.)

Alcohol is without doubt one of the most addictive chemicals on God's earth. For some people, alcohol is more addictive than is caffeine, codeine, cocaine or heroin. Because of its addictive effects, wine easily violates Principle III. Because processing is necessary to add the percentages of alcohol present in modern wines, they

Russell's Milk Preferences From Greatest to Least

1. Raw, organic clean milk from cows that are free from hormone injections, antibiotic regimes and concentrated pesticide sprays. Raw milk will spoil rapidly if warmed.

2. Pasteurized, nonhomogenized milk.

3. Pasteurized and skimmed milk.

4. Skimmed milk.

5. Pasteurized and homogenized milk.

A final word about milk: milk is like meat —you don't need a lot of it and you can live without it.

violate Principle II. And because of its effect on the brain and muscular control, alcohol may be the number one destroyer of health in the world. Therefore, I would recommend little or no routine use of alcoholic products.

In evaluating wine on principle, I believe that water or freshly squeezed fruit juices or low alcoholic wines are what God intended for us, particularly for health.

What About Other Beverages?

The implications other beverages have for our health depend on what is dissolved in the great basic beverage— water.

Coffee has been implicated in causing cancer of the pancreas, and in raising cholesterol. More careful research indicates that though boiled coffee appears to have some of these harmful effects, filtered coffee shows no correlation with them.

Coffee can, however, easily violate Principle III by causing addiction. Caffeine is one of the world's most psychoactive drugs. Once we start

using it, it is hard to escape. Caffeine is found in coffee (40-150 mgs. per cup), soft drinks (50-74 mgs.), tea (20-50 mgs.), chocolate (5-29 mgs.) and in some medications.

Colas are also suspect. Coca-Cola was first marketed in 1886, by a pharmacist in Atlanta, Georgia, as the drink that had a kick, but that had none of alcohol's harmful effects. The drink was an immediate hit. The pharmacist's customers became so loyal that they would take their Coke with them everywhere. Of course, it turned out that the key ingredient was cocaine! The key to Coca-Cola's early success was addiction.

Although the cocaine was outlawed in 1900, most colas and other soft drinks are still addictive. Rather than cocaine, they are loaded with sugar, caffeine and sodium. One Coke has the equivalent sugar content of 10 to 12 apples or 15 feet of sugar cane. The caffeine in a single bottle of some soda pop equals that of a cup of coffee.

Colas also have additional additives such as phosphorous, which decreases the absorption of needed calcium and diminishes some nerve function. It also causes the kidneys to excrete excessive calcium,[19] which affects bones; iron, which is needed for

blood; and magnesium,[20] which affects muscle contractibility and cellular functions.

Diet colas have been shown to contain six times as much sodium as regular soda does—both contain too much sodium.

In Conclusion

Recommendation:

If you want to improve your health or prevent afflictions, you need only to follow a simple course revealed by your Designer's own Word.

Drink water, juice and milk as near to their designed state as possible. A squeeze of lemon, lime or some honey will add variety to water.

Juices made directly from fruits are already highly purified because they have been filtered through the plant— they are great. Pure water added to fruit-juice concentrates is also good, but remember that tap water may contain chlorine or other chemicals— a violation of Principle II.

Enjoy clean, chemical-free milk. It is hard to get, but your search will be rewarded with good health. Grade A pasteurized milk is heated to drop the bacteria count to less than 25,000 per cubic centimeter of milk. Certified raw milk is required to have a bacterial count of less than 10,000 per cubic centimeter of milk. After a few days of cold storage, clean milks, whether pasteurized or raw, yield equal counts of bacteria.

Avoid chemicalized tap water, coffee and tea.

Avoid alcoholic beverages.

Avoid chemicalized, highly sugared, caffeinated or artificially sweetened drinks.

Remember that water transports nutrients to our cells in beverages. We need plenty of it. It is the best solvent for all the products of digestion. It removes waste. It regulates body temperature. It is the elixir of life—but it can poison you with what is dissolved in it.

Appendix 1.

Answers to "Check Your Health IQ"

(See page 6)

1. Fiber = +. Fiber is good for your health. The fiber we get naturally in vegetables, fruits and seeds is always covered with great nutrients that protect us from many harmful substances and diseases. Fiber is also necessary because it "sweeps" the digestive tract clean.

2. Nuts = +. Nuts contain wonderful oils and fats that are essential for your health. In addition, they have the ideal amino acids for building protein and enzymes. Nuts contain only a small amount of complex carbohydrates and essentially no simple carbohydrates. Processing (adding animal fat and/or too much salt) is about the only thing that would make nuts less healthful.

3. Whole-grain cereals = +. Whole-grain cereals are good, but some may contain too much sugar. Some whole-grain cereals such as granola have a sugar content as high as 60 percent. Watch for this. If you have to add sweeteners to your cereal, use a small amount of juice.

4. Sunlight = +. Sunlight is good. Sunlight activates many ingredients in our cells that come from whole foods. Vitamin D, anticancer, antiviral, antiarthritic and insect repellent components are formed from sunlight. Without whole food, sunshine's ultraviolet light has a greater chance of damaging the skin.

5. Swordfish = +. Biblically, this fish is good for your health in that it does have scales and fins. It also has a good supply of the healthy 3-omega fatty acids.

6. Marriage = +. Studies have shown that marriage is beneficial to a person's longevity. In the marriage relationship, the husband seems to gain the most as far as longevity is concerned. Except in unusual circumstances, staying married is definitely the healthiest thing you can do for yourself. Often you can do nothing about being widowed or separated. This is not the end of the world. Many things can improve your longevity and joy of living in both the widowed and separated circumstance. Probably the most important thing to remember is that God promises through the Holy Spirit to be your Counselor and Companion. Many have rested in this relationship and flourished.

7. "Type A" personality = 0 (neutral). Longevity studies on heart and cancer patients fail to demonstrate any difference between "type A" and "type B" personalities. Caregivers had generally thought that "type A" personalities were more apt to have heart disease, ulcers and other diseases. This has not been proven to be true. Often the "type A" personality will do better in recovery because the personality lends to following the doctor's orders explicitly.[1]

8. "Type B" personality = 0 (neutral; see **number 7**).

***9. Bitterness = –.** The only personality trait that proves to be harmful for our health is bitterness. The origin of bitterness and hostility is usually a lack of forgiveness.

Peter asked Jesus how often we should forgive someone who offends us. "Is seven times enough?" he asked, in effect. Jesus' response was, "seventy-seven times" (Matt. 18:21,22). In other words, we are to forgive indefinitely. It is healthful to forgive, and it is harmful to hold a grudge. Remember the Scripture, "Vengeance is mine;...saith the Lord" (Rom. 12:19, KJV). Dr. Dean Ornish, famous for his methods of reversing vascular disease, agrees that the "most toxic" personality traits to the heart are hostility and cynicism.[2]

10. Olive oil = +. Years ago, when olive oil was considered bad for health, a study of seven countries showed that the citizens of Sicily had more fat in their diets than all the other countries studied. Yet the Sicilians had less vascular heart disease and other health problems. The primary source of fat they were eating was olive oil. More studies have shown many benefits of olive oil.

11. Butter = +. Butter is a saturated fatty acid and contains cholesterol, a fact that has resulted in butter's being condemned by most nutritionists. However, butter is a good food, when eaten in moderation. Butter does not raise the levels of cholesterol or harmful fats in the blood. Both olive oil and butter are digested by humans in a way similar to the way complex carbohydrates are digested. Complex carbohydrates are also healthful.

12. Margarine = –. The processing (hydrogenation of oils) of margarine forms trans fatty acids. This form of fatty acids represent a big problem for our cells. It increases vascular disease and cancers. It also elevates the bad cholesterol and triglycerides in our blood.[3] Considering all the negative aspects of margarine, butter would be a better choice.

***13. Safe sex with a condom = –.** It is not good for your health. The chondyloma virus, which is one of about 30 known venereal diseases, is passed in 100 percent of sexual contacts when one partner is infected even when a condom is used.

14. Wine = –. In general, I would rate

wine as a negative. Wine has at least two unhealthful ingredients: sulfites and alcohol. The University of Wisconsin recently reported that bioflavins in wine are good for the vessels and for the heart. That is true; but the wine industry and its advertisers make their reports sound as though bioflavins are found only in wine. The fact is they are found in higher concentrations in juices, fruit and vegetables than in wines.

Also, alcohol damages all cells. Even a small amount of alcohol weakens the heart muscle. Abstinence from alcohol strengthens the heart's contraction ability unless permanent damage has already been done. The alcohol concentrations in wine are increased by adding sugar to juice before fermenting.

15. Rest = +. Scripture commands one day of rest a week. You probably will get more done in six days of hard work preceded by a day off than you can possibly get done on a nonstop schedule. Efficiency at work is more valuable than time spent at work. Don't think that because God commanded one day of rest a week that you need more time off. It may be nice if you can get it. Sleep is also positively related to physical and mental health. Again, however, be warned: balance is important:

> *How long will you lie there, you sluggard? When will you get up from your sleep? A little sleep, a little slumber, a little folding of the hands to rest—and poverty will come on you like a bandit and scarcity like an armed man* (Prov. 6:9-11).

*16. Same-gender sex = –. Same-gender sex is devastating to your health. See chapter 4.

17. Live fruits = +. "Live" (or fresh) fruits are those whose seeds are still viable or able to reproduce. Chemicals, radiation and other processing destroy the seed's ability to reproduce. In general, fruits are excellent for your health, but they are best for you when eaten "live." I still would heartily recommended "raw" fruit, even though now fruits can be radiated and chemicalized to increase storage life, and this is detrimental to their bio-usefulness.

18. Avocados = +. Surprise! In my opinion avocados are good for your health. It is true they do contain fat, but these are fats that heal rather than fats that kill. Avocados contain fiber and nutrients. They are a well-designed food, when eaten in moderation. Enjoy!

19. Sweating from labor = +. This is not referring to the delivery of a baby. In this case, "sweating" refers to physical labor such as working as a roofer or furniture mover. Physical exercise and eating good nutrients go hand in hand.

20. Sprouts = +. Because sprouts are growing and alive, many people think they are especially good for you. Alfalfa seeds, mung beans and so on can be grown in a glass jar for three or four days and used in salads or on sandwiches. Sprouts can be bought in the produce section of your grocery store, and are an easy and painless way to get good nutrients.

21. Live vegetables = +. Live vegetables are much like sprouts or seeds. They are either growing or have the potential to grow. Buying green beans in the produce section is better than buying canned beans. Be aware that some vegetables may be radiated or chemically altered.

22. Beef = +. Surprise again! Beef is healthy if you eat only the flesh and not the cover fat or blood. Overfeeding and overmedicating with hormones and antibiotics can change the product. The healthy 3-omega fatty acids are altered, causing the beef to be unhealthy. Chemicals in the animal's flesh may have other detrimental effects. I will admit that it's hard to tell which cows have been overmedicated when you are strolling through the meat department of your local grocery store! If possible, find chemical-free, grass-fed beef. Many caregivers classify beef and pork together because they are both red meat. Actually, they are as different as night from day. The Bible describes beef as clean and pork as unclean (see number 23). Other KJV words for "cow" are "ox," "oxen," "heifer," "bullock" and "cow."

*23. Pork = –. Scripture mentions pork many times and always having a negative connotation. The pig's flesh is described as "putrid," "filthy" or "unclean." Humans classify pork as a red meat, but the Bible groups pork with blood, bowel movements, road kill, buzzards, snakes, rats and roaches. In my opinion, eating pork may be the most damaging item on this list. Give yourself five points for getting this one right.

24. Homogenized milk = –. The main reason milk is homogenized is so its butterfat does not float to the top. This cosmetic effect is costly for health reasons. The large fat globules are broken down into tiny globules. When broken down (homogenized), these smaller globules can enter the arteries and cause ulcers and plaques. Scripture mentions milk as an item intended for food. The milk mentioned in the Bible did not derive from animals that were given hormones, antibiotics and other chemicals. Sources of raw, clean, chemical-free milk are available, but they are difficult to find.

25. Soft drinks = –. Americans consume huge amounts of soft drinks. The phosphorus in cola blocks the absorption of valuable nutrients such as calcium, magnesium and manganese. Drinking soft drinks would be okay occasionally, but not daily. Diet drinks are no improvement.

26. Same-spouse sex = +. Same-spouse sex is designed and approved of by God for pleasure and procreation. In today's society, sex should be considered a high risk. The only people who can enjoy "safe sex" are those in a lifelong, monogamous relationship. Enjoy.

27. Juice = +. All juices are good, but freshly squeezed juices have many additional benefits compared to those made from concentrate. Try diluting the juice to keep from absorbing such a high concentration of simple sugar. Sparkling water may be added to the juices to make them more attractive. "Smoothie" recipes are easy to find. Blend juices, honey, frozen fruits, cinnamon and ice for a healthful and tasty treat.

*28. Smoking = –. If you are a smoker, your best protection is to eat large amounts of fresh vegetables, fruits and grains. Another protection might be periodic abstinence. For those who cannot or will not quit using tobacco, a better choice would be chemical-free, organic tobacco. Tobacco plants are heavily sprayed and many chemicals are added during processing. Your best choice remains to quit!

29. Cover fat on meat = –. Scripture states that we should not eat the fat of the ox, sheep or goat. This is the layer of fat between the muscle and the skin. Fat that covers the internal organs should be avoided as well. Caregivers have learned that cancer, hardening of the arteries and other health problems are present in people who eat this kind of fat. Remember that although oxen, sheep and goats are clearly declared to be clean, certain tissues in these animals, such as blood and fat, Scripture declares unclean. This fat is often added to ground beef and other products, including wieners and sausage.

30. Anger = 0 (neutral). This is one of our designed emotions. Certainly we have examples of anger demonstrated by both our Creator and by Jesus. Anger, to be healthy, must be controlled. Some evil in this world needs our wrath poured out on it. Anger can serve to control evil. "Be...angry, and sin not" (Eph. 4:26, KJV).

31. Blond hair = 0 (neutral). The color of your hair doesn't have any affect on your health. This item was a "gimme" in the quiz for those who have not scored well so far.

32. Sunglasses = –. Sunglasses are good news/bad news. Sunglasses that block ultraviolet rays can protect the eyes, but others do not. They can actually inhibit the normal contraction of the pupil when exposed to light. That just allows more of the harmful rays into the eye. Also, some research shows that glasses advertised as blocking ultraviolet rays still allow "a" rays to enter the eye (see question 4, appendix 2).

*33. Shellfish = –. The Creator defines shellfish as putrid and foul. Shellfish are designed to clean lakes, ponds, oceans and rivers of harmful chemical and bacterial pollution. Many deaths and epidemics can be traced to contaminated shellfish. See also pork, number 23 in this quiz, and chapter 8 about meats.

34. Prayer = +. Prayer is amazing. Even secular researchers agree that prayer has a beneficial effect on your health.

*35. Alcohol = –. Research and experience have proven overwhelmingly that alcohol is harmful for your health. Many in this world worship alcohol. It is their god. Don't be fooled by isolated reports touting supposed benefits. (See also number 14.)

36. Fasting = +. Scripture tells us that fasting is a "wellspring of health." See chapter 5.

37. Forgiveness - +. Many psychiatrists who have studied the effect of forgiveness on our spirits, minds and bodies are impressed by its remarkable healing effects. The cornerstone of good mental health is based on forgiveness.

38. Breast feeding = +. In spite of the multitude of known benefits, it is amazing how few mothers breast-feed their babies. It is a valuable investment.

39. Large-mouth bass = +. This fish has both scales and fins, so it is good.

40. Catfish = –. This fish was designed with no scales; therefore it is unclean. The decision not to eat catfish and other scavengers should be an easy one. My motive is to encourage you to enjoy the good things God has created for food. He wrote the Book, and He does command you to avoid certain specific animals. See chapter 8.

41. Smiling = +. Both the giver and the receiver of a smile benefit through the release of prostaglandins. These substances help balance the hormonal functions of the body. An employee in my hospital whose nickname is "Smiley" encourages us with her happy spirit. I have noticed that many technicians who have winning smiles can change a cantankerous patient into a compliant one.

*42. Promiscuity = –. Promiscuity promotes almost as many health hazards as do other sexual defilements of the body. It is devastating spiritually, mentally and physically.

43. Hot dogs = –. My one-time favorite now ranks at the bottom of the list. Hot dogs are composed of unclean flesh, and contain a saturated fat content of up to 70 percent. They can be composed of lots of things you really don't want to know about—animal skin, hair and so on.

44. Divorce = –. Many studies have shown that divorce is bad for your health. (Sometimes it also indicates bad theology, or none at all, because God said, "I hate divorce" [Mal. 2:16]. This of course doesn't mean that divorce is the unforgivable sin, or that it isn't sometimes a tragic necessity; and in any case our focus here is on physical health.)

Researchers Thomas Holmes and Richard Rahe developed a scale of "stressors" that typically set us up for emotional and/or physical illness. Divorce was second only to the death of a spouse in its damaging effect on the whole person.[4]

Appendix 2
Frequently Asked Questions

When I conduct seminars or speak about eating biblically, I'm asked all kinds of questions. I hope answering them in this chapter will speak to questions you might also be asking.

1. If the ways of the Creator are best for our health, what about the harmful effects of sunlight on the skin?

The harmful effects of sunshine include burns, skin cancer and premature aging. Actually, the food (*bromah*) God created for humans is loaded with ingredients to turn the sun's energy into vitamin D and other vital nutrients. Foods also have ingredients that block the harmful effects of ultraviolet rays.

The phytochemicals in foods do much more than just protect our skin from ultraviolet rays. Activated by the sunlight, they also produce antiviral, antibacterial, and anticancer components, as well as pest repellents.[1] If we obeyed Principle II and ate unprocessed food (*bromah*), most premature skin aging, blisters, cancer and so on would not be a problem. The ingredients found in commercial sunscreens are also found naturally in *bromah* food. Our heavenly Father, not the pharmaceutical industry, has given us the raw materials in food that is used to make sunscreen.

Remember also Principle III, and don't worship the sun. Jesus said:

I am the light of the world. Whoever follows me will never walk in darkness, but will have the light of life (John 8:12).

All of us are tempted to worship the Creation rather than the Creator.

2. If God created sunlight, why does it damage our eyes?

God saw that the light was good (Gen. 1:4).

Sunshine is implicated in both macular degeneration (AMC) and cataracts, which are diseases that can cause blindness, particularly in the elderly. AMC affects the center of the retina and is the leading cause of blindness in people over 65. Cataracts are the result of clouding in the lens of the eye. Fortunately, sight is fairly easily restored by replacing the clouded lens with a plastic lens.

The *University of California-Berkeley Letter* (January 1988) reviewed the current research about preventing these causes of blindness, analyzing the effects of multiple vitamins, minerals and phytochemicals. Although researchers gave a guarded recommendation for vitamin supplements, they enthusiastically supported the concept that the major key to prevention was a diet rich in fruits, whole grains and vegetables.

Many ophthalmologists, including Dr. Jerald Tennant of the Dallas Eye Institute, maintain that the progression of both of these eye diseases can be halted if a nutrient-rich formula of foods (*bromah*), plus natural supplements, are ingested regularly. He recommends the supplements be made from grains, sprouts and vegetables such as barley or carrots.

3. How can some scientists maintain that blind, random chance produced a seeing eye?

Charles Darwin deserves to be quoted about this:

To suppose that the eye with all its inimitable contrivances for adjusting the focus to different distances, for admitting different amounts of light, and for the correction of spherical and chromatic aberrations, could have been formed by natural selection, seems, I freely confess, absurd in the highest degree.[2]

4. Are sunglasses good for you?

Darwin's wonder at the eye's ability to admit different amounts of light is important in giving the best answer concerning the value of sunglasses.

The visible light rays do not damage the lens or the macula of our eyes; the ultraviolet rays do. Sunglasses block the visible spectrum of light from entering the pupil of the eye. Normally the pupil contracts to a very small size when exposed to light; but dark glasses negate this contraction. When we wear sunglasses that do not block the ultraviolet rays but merely open up the pupil in the eye, we allow more ultraviolet light to enter them.

Ultraviolet (UV) light interacts with human tissue biochemically. Blocking UV rays from entering the eyes will help prevent cataracts and macular degeneration in much the same way that suntan lotion prevents sunburn.

But there is one big problem. According to Dr. Tennant, the UV glasses we buy over the counter block only ultraviolet-b and ultraviolet-c rays.[3] The UV-a rays that are not filtered out do the most damage to the eyes. It is unbelievable how often our best ideas, such as sunglasses, do more harm than good.

Our best options:

1. Go without sunglasses; let our eyes constrict so that very little of the damaging light gets into our eyes.

2. Eat mostly whole food—*bromah*—containing phytochemicals that will protect our eyes much like they protect the skin from UV rays.

3. Buy special glasses that specifically block UV-a rays (as well as the b and c rays).[4]

5. What about picante or salsa?

These tomato-based sauces have become the number one best-seller of all condiments. The primary component of picante is tomatoes. The more we learn about tomatoes, the more valuable we think they are. One ingredient in tomatoes is lycopenes, a potent antioxidant. They are extremely effective at protecting cells from all kinds of insults, infections, chemical, heat and radiation. Lycopenes are not harmed by heat, and are stable in all kinds of products. The mobile elderly invariably have higher blood levels of lycopenes than the more infirmed. Cancer patients have lower levels of lycopenes than noncancer patients. *Enjoy* picante!

6. How do I regain the health I've lost from improper eating habits?

If you have lived an "unclean" lifestyle, be honest and say so. If your lifestyle has been "un*lean*," confess that, too. Pray something like this: "I have been deceived, fooled and unmindful of treating my body as a temple of the Holy Spirit (see 1 Cor. 6:19). Creator,

Holy Spirit, lead me and heal me and help me to discipline my body. Take control of this part of my life."

Memorize 1 Corinthians 10:13:
No temptation has seized you except what is common to man. And God is faithful; he will not let you be tempted beyond what you can bear. But when you are tempted, he will also provide a way out so that you can stand up under it.

Discuss your intentions with your spouse and friends. Ask their help. Encourage them to join you in your commitment, but don't require them to eat your way. Your commitment should be between you and your Designer. Don't check up on others; you have a big enough job just checking on yourself.

Memorize The Three Principles. Evaluate everything you eat or do with these in mind. When questions arise, ask your Instructor, the Holy Spirit.

Don't bother to argue. When offered something harmful, such as catfish, pork, shellfish and other scavengers, just say, "crocodile gizzards" just don't agree with me. Smile, but don't join them in eating what you know God did not create for food.

Then eat—with enthusiasm—a lot of the right kinds of unprocessed food—food that is designed for you. These words will start creeping into your vocabulary: "I feel good."

Set up a point system for everyone in your family, awarding points for eating God's way. Keep a weekly score. Award a prize number to the latest winner. A $20 bill. A toy. A massage. Whatever.

Here is how to keep score. Every fresh vegetable, fruit or tablespoon of whole grain or nuts (raw) = 10 points. Whole grain products = 5 points. Maximum score = 20 points for any one item.

Any item of Principle I food at a meal = 5 points, even if it is processed. Any white flour, white sugar or processed oil = –10 points. Any unclean food = –30 points.

A 15- to 20-hour fast with water or juice once a week = 50 points.

Make up your own rules to make it more fun.

After one week, set a daily goal for each participant. It is certainly a good idea to have the prize be valuable, because if you are responsible for paying their doctor bills you will more than likely be saving plenty.

By contrast, the worst thing you can do for your health is to go the opposite of God's way. Eating the things not created for food is foolish!

If others are interested, form a support club. It can be easier and more fun. Adapting AA's 12 steps will help. Be sure to use Scripture as much as possible.

7. If I exercise, do I still need to eat right?
Yes.

It is my belief that we need enough exercise to work up a sweat six days a week. It is hard to find enough time, but it is worth it. Do it. The Bible says, "by the sweat of your brow you will eat your food" (Gen. 3:19). Because most of us no longer toil in the fields for our food, physical exercise should be substituted.

Several hormones formed naturally in our bodies are apparently enhanced by exercise. Exercise also balances the function of these hormones. This balancing effect produces higher levels of cytokines—substances that improve the immune system.

The benefits of exercise and good nutrition go hand in hand. In one study, exercisers ate approximately the same amount of calories as those who were sedentary. The exercisers had a higher intake of every vitamin, mineral and amino acid. They also consumed far less coffee, alcohol, tobacco, sugar and naked calories. If you consider this advice, it is easy to see that exercise can often replace tranquilizers[5] and improve health in general.

Finally (and this should get your attention), exercise has been shown to drop the death rate sixfold in men ages 50 to 54.[6]

Remember The Third Principle, however, and don't worship exercise, or overdo it. Many do, to their detriment. Don't think you have to be an Olympian. Many healthful activities can strengthen your whole system.

8. Is eating totally healthy really possible on a limited budget?
Yes!

One trip to the doctor can cost more than a six-month supply of grains, beans, peas, nuts, onions, potatoes and garlic. Twenty-five pounds of organic grain will last six months, and costs only $15.

Breads, soups, sprouts, casseroles and so on can be prepared on a limited budget, and they are extremely healthful. Remember that in most cultures the wealthy often eat the poorest food. Processed foods are expensive compared to whole foods.

9. What about limited time?
Start spending less time cooking, and begin eating more meals composed of raw fruits and vegetables. Even grains and nuts are great for you raw. Remember that Jesus and His disciples ate raw grain while walking from one place to another. Eating right can save time.

Speaking of saving time, fasting can add hours to an otherwise busy day simply by saving the time you would ordinarily spend preparing and eating food.

The combination of fasting, then eating fruits, veggies and whole grains, is great for both time and health. Remember that animals and humans who eat foods containing very low caloric content have the greatest longevity. So don't worry if you miss a meal once in a while.

Co-op cooking and buying is another way many have succeeded in saving time and money. Remember also that food is a blessing. It is very important. Enjoy!

10. Where can I find pure food?
At our house, the best source of organic, dehydrated broccoli at a great price is found in a crack in our kitchen table. We discovered this "hidey hole" when our second son left for college. You can probably find better sources—maybe even in your own kitchen! Many grocery stores now provide excellent sources of breads, vegetables and fruits. Health-food stores are also found in many small towns. Mail-order catalogs for supplies are available. The best source of pure food is your own garden.

11. What about the pesticides on produce?
Pesticide- and chemical-free produce are bargains at any price, but other produce can still have great value for your health. Pesticides have to be detoxified by our bodies when they are ingested on the food we eat. In addition, fiber in the system clings to many harmful chemicals, taking them out with fecal waste. Detoxification requires many vitamins, minerals and other nutrients, and interestingly these detoxifying nutrients are found in highest concentrations in produce. Wash the produce well before eating. The optimal plan would be to buy organically grown fruits and vegetables.

12. Is holistic medicine best?
No! Yes! The term "holistic" refers to the body, mind and spirit. The spiritual aspects of health are in the supernatural realm. Although that sounds great, many in the field of holistic medicine are not seeking the Creator's supernatural help. Be aware that according to the Bible, evil spirits also have power to heal. They will deceive you and make you look ridiculous, possibly robbing you of your health.

Some holistic healers follow New Age teaching, which includes a lot of things that are in fact good for health. But be careful! Many New Agers worship the Creation rather than the Creator. They claim that humankind is evolving into gods or higher spiritual beings. Their philosophy often sounds good, but remember that God creates and Satan imitates. Can Satan fool us? Sure.

Compare any health plan with God's Word.

13. What are "naked calories"?

Proteins, carbohydrates and lipids contain calories. In God's original design, these substances are "covered" with nutrients. The processing that yields white flour, sugar and clear oils also removes this "clothing" of nutrients, leaving only "naked calories." Naked calories can add weight and cause various nutrient imbalances while providing no benefits. They make us disinterested in true *bromah* while leaving us hungry.

14. What do you eat at a Chinese restaurant?

I basically don't eat much meat at any restaurant because I can get chemical-free meat at home. At a Chinese restaurant I might order some vegetable chow mein or chop suey, instructing them to please leave off monosodium glutamate. Also I like mine hot and spicy.

I ask them to cut the oil by 50 percent, unless they are using olive oil. A few treasures are to be found in almost all eating places.

15. Are vitamins necessary?

Food is your best medicine, and food is also your best supplement. If you could eat fresh, chemical-free foods regularly, vitamins and minerals would serve no purpose. I believe they are necessary for most of us, however, because we simply don't eat enough healthful foods. Many philosophies or plans are believed about supplements. Choose one based on your own needs and let the supplement be as near to a designed food as possible. "Natural" vitamins probably are best because they will have many other associated food factors attached to them. Evaluate all supplement plans by The Three Principles. I take vitamins and some herbal preparations as well, but I would not ask you to do it my way. Ask your health consultant.

16. If I pray over my food, doesn't that make it okay?

No! First Timothy 4:4,5 does say:

For everything God created is good, and nothing is to be rejected if it is received with thanksgiving, because it is consecrated by the word of God and prayer.

Paul was obviously speaking of things God created for food. Paul also refers to the Word of God for consecrating the food being blessed. Actually, Paul was considering a heresy that maintained that all meat was "carnal"—not with the legitimate distinction between clean (wholesome) and unclean meats.

17. How can I control obesity?

Many books have been written about obesity. Although eating according to God's design may not be an adequate solution by itself, it certainly is foundational. It is a simple concept that if we are eating nutritious food only, our weight will settle at our normal, most ideal poundage and we can throw the scales away.

For those seeking practical advice, the best information and recommendations I have seen are contained in a pamphlet called "38 Practical Ways to Achieve Your Proper Weight" (Basic Care Program, Box 3113, Oak Brook, Ill. 60522-3113, phone (708) 323-9800).

18. What personalities are more likely to get sick?

For years, studies have suggested that the "type A" personality—the hard-driving type—is more frequently subject to heart attacks, mental illness and so on. More recent studies about personality traits, however, have shown that type A and type B personalities are equal as far as the occurrence and progression of disease is concerned.[7] The only personality trait that has been shown to be detrimental to health is hostility or bitterness.[8] The root cause of bitterness is holding a grudge. Being unforgiving and seeking to avenge a wrong committed against you are both spiritually and physically unhealthful.

19. You said that doing things by The Three Principles would prevent the leading causes of death. What about accidents?

In l986, accidents were the fourth leading cause of death in the United States. They certainly are one of the major causes of hospitalization. Statistics tell us, however, that the majority of deaths are related to alcohol and drugs. This is true at home, or when traveling by water, air, rail or highway. Certainly this is an example of consuming things that were not intended for food (Principles I and II); and many drug and alcohol related deaths are the result of addictions, or the violation of Principle III. Forty percent of our population will at some time in life be involved in an accident caused by someone drinking.

20. How can an athletic team or an individual reach maximum performance?

The following disciplines are keys for top performance:

1. Drink plenty of clean water.
2. Avoid potentially addictive substances.
3. Eat fresh, whole foods.
4. Eat clean meat occasionally.
5. Get plenty of exercise.
6. Practice good hygiene.
7. Fast occasionally.
8. Pray.

9. Wear 100 percent cotton cloth or 100 percent wool clothing against your skin.

Guess what? All of this advice came from the Bible and was given to the Israelite armies of the Old Testament when they were the all-time greatest "against all odds" winners. They seemed to have supernatural fighting skills, particularly when they were obedient to God. They failed dismally when they did not follow God's direction. They learned that obedience was better than sacrifice. They learned:

Since the Lord your God walks in the midst of your camp to deliver you and to defeat your enemies before you, therefore your camp must be holy; and He must not see anything indecent among you lest He turn away from you (Deut. 23:14, NASB).

The soldiers were to follow the sanitary rules for Israel's military camp. Similar rules for the people in general are found in Leviticus 15.

21. What mistakes have you made with The Three Principles?

For some time, I refused to look at Principle II regarding milk and oils. For the first five years I studied all this, I was stubborn and refused to read about milk. Then it took some time for me to decide to seek clean, unprocessed milk instead of drinking conventional pasteurized milk. Later we enjoyed raw, certified milk, but since it is no longer available in our area I basically don't drink much milk anymore.

Because the oils derived from such foods as corn and other vegetables are designed by God, I was sure that polyunsaturated oil was safe and healthful. However, I mistakenly ignored the information about how much processing went into oil's formation. I did realize early that margarine was ridiculous, but it took a lot of information, both subtle and obvious, to force me to look at my own Principle II and say that most oils had been tampered with far too much.

One reason I finally looked at the evidence was that I had a blood vessel narrow to the point of stopping flow, even while I was eating right in some areas. I thoroughly reevaluated every food item. Now I seriously try to limit my oil intake to olive oil (virgin) or butter.

22. What suggestions do you have for a meat-and-potato man who is addicted to salt, sugar, caffeine, fat and scavengers?

Search for clean, chemical-free meat.

Load your potato with healthful stuff—picante, butter or vegetables.

Pop some popcorn in olive oil or butter, and salt it lightly with sea salt.

Stir-fry some vegetables in olive oil. Add hot sauce. That is macho. You are the toughest if you add enough hot sauce to sweat.

Cut fresh avocado slices with lemon juice brushed on to taste. Avocado is healthful fat.

Bake some wheat sticks and dip them in olive oil mixed with salt-free herbal seasonings.

Add spices to anything.

Put a lot of onions or garlic on everything.

23. Don't your genes determine how long you will live?

During an interview, a gentleman who was 109 years old was asked to identify the key to his longevity. He answered, "The reason I have lived so long is that I quit smoking and drinking when I was 103." I hope he was lying, but nearly everyone has at least one acquaintance who lived to an old age, but broke all of the rules. Scripture does speak of some who have a particularly strong constitution and will live longer (see Ps. 90:9,10). Is there is any advantage to a longer life if misery could have been avoided, and was not?

24. Is there any way to smoke and still live a normal, full life?

Probably not. Your only chance would be to go on a Genesis 1:29 diet, consuming huge amounts of fresh vegetables, herbs and seeds. The best way is still to stop. Period. Studies do show some protective effect in smokers for cancer and strokes when they eat a lot of *bromah*—things God created for food.

25. What about hormones (melotonin, estrogen, testosterone and DHEA) for aging, sleep, antioxidant action and so on?

The risk of ingesting these products regularly is not known. The body's production of these hormones and others is known to be enhanced by—guess what? Real food. For melotonin it is rice, sweet corn, tomatoes, ginger, oats, bananas and barley. Seeds enhance estrogen production and actually supply estrogen in an unusual but absolutely natural form.

26. What about prayer for healing and health?

Scripturally, this appears to be the beginning of recovery. We need to pray personally, with family, with a friend, with an elder (see Jas. 5:14). On a personal level, we should not only ask for healing, but also for help in understanding the cause of our illness—whether it might be (1) a sickness unto death, in which case we should thank the Lord that He is calling us home; (2) for the glory of God—to show His power, love or design; (3) the result of bad choices or wrongdoing, in which case we should pray that God will teach us so that we can repent and then go the opposite way; (4) the result of someone else's mistake, in which case we should ask for wisdom to protect ourselves and our families from the careless ways of the world.

27. What if my prayers are unanswered?

Start practicing The Three Principles.

28. Why are some saints' prayers unanswered?

God is omnipotent. He answers your prayers any way He chooses. His promises can be relied on for healing of many illnesses. Occasionally, He chooses to glorify Himself with a miraculous healing. I have neither heard of nor yet found a technique to manipulate Him into action. Often His actions appear limited or oddly specific as if to teach one individual or small group of His power. Be careful: Satan and his demons can deceive people with their own apparent miracles, and they even have some power to temporarily improve health.

Remember also that a part of the curse of the Fall is the thorn. Paul had one. So carry on.

29. How do The Three Principles help hypertension?

An article in *The Journal of Hypertension* related that just adding some fiber to the diets of randomly selected patients resulted in significant lowering of the diastolic blood pressure.[9] Other research has shown even more pronounced effects when God-designed food is primarily eaten after fasting.

30. You seem to be indicating that fasting and The Three Principles will help most diseases. Are any measurable laboratory changes (in blood or urine tests) found once these lifestyle changes take place?

Nearly every aspect of health has been shown to improve by proper diet and appropriate fasting. My point is well illustrated by a report showing that 14 parameters indicating rheumatoid arthritis improved in a group of patients who were "treated" with a combination of fasting and an essentially vegetarian diet. On the other hand, none of these 14 parameters improved in those who returned to a regular diet.[10]

31. Who is the devil? What does he do?

His name "Satan" means adversary; and the Bible describes him as a deceiver and a liar, the opponent of all that is good:

There is no truth in him. When he lies, he speaks his native language, for he is a liar and the father of lies (John 8:44).

The relevance of the devil to the issues in this book is that he has deceived us into accepting the lies of the world regarding what we eat, while we should be adhering to the truth of God's Word. This makes it all important to check everything you read—including this book—by the Word.

Have I ever been deceived? Is a bluebird blue?

32. Do you have any study tips for the New Testament concerning your message?

Look up the following Greek words from *Strong's Exhaustive Concordance* when studying any difficult text about eating. Look up the references in your Bible to see how the Greek word is used.

1. *bromah*—Greek bro'-mah; food (lit. or fig.), especially articles allowed or forbidden by the Jewish law—meat, victuals. Used 13 times in the New Testament.

2. *trophe*—food, rations, vegetables.

3. *koinos*—common, shared by all or defiled. Acts 10:14,15; 11:8,9; Romans 14:14.

4. *akethartos*—foul, unclean, impure. Acts 10:14,28; 11:8.

5. *nomos*—law—regulations given through Moses or the Gospels.

6. *paradosis*—Jewish traditions added to God's law.

7. *katharizo*—to make clean, pure or holy.

8. *hagios*—sacred, pure, blameless. First Timothy 1:8: "We know that the law [*nomos*-law: regulations given through Moses or the Gospels] is good if one uses it properly." Christ and the authors of the New Testament objected and frequently instructed against the use of the Law for salvation. The Law is otherwise highly valued.

Appendix 3

How to Begin a Relationship with Your Creator

The Difference Biblical Faith Makes

A tremendous advantage of accepting the historical evidence offered by the Bible is that it describes how the Creator graciously reveals Himself to us.

He reveals Himself through creation, or nature, its marvelous design pointing to a Designer.

He reveals Himself through history, as in the birth of His Son, Jesus Christ.

He also reveals Himself through a special text we call the Bible.

The primary message of the Bible is that we can have a personal relationship with the Creator—a relationship called "salvation." We need this relationship because it substitutes His sinlessness for our sinful nature. Otherwise, we truly have no hope.

The way I like to envision our sin nature is to consider how we just naturally like to do things our own way. I believe we are born with this trait, as can be evidenced in a small baby who wants things done strictly according to his or her selfish impulses.

Every book of the Bible tells us that this nature, which is inherited from Adam, separates us from God, and that innocent blood must be shed for the remission of the sins that abound in this sin nature.

The Bible is filled with illustrations of this truth. The blood of an innocent animal was shed for Adam and Eve to cover themselves with skins after the original sin. Centuries later, Abraham was willing to sacrifice his innocent son, Isaac, as a type of the Messiah who would one day actually be sacrificed for the sins of all humankind. The law of Moses dictated that innocent animals were to be slain to cover humans' sins.

Additionally, hundreds of prophecies throughout the Bible told that one day the Messiah, the Christ, would come and offer the perfect sacrifice. This would be God Himself, in the person of Jesus Christ.

Of course what God creates, Satan counterfeits or imitates. He has caused many variations of this message to deceive us. Counterfeit religions have been created that involve the worship of man or nature—the sun, moon, stars, even animals. Deceitful sacrifices have also involved the sacrifice of children—actual sacrifices, not just tests, as in the case of Abraham and his son, Isaac.

This is why it is extremely important to be guided in our search for the Creator by His Word, the Bible. The basic biblical way to establish a relationship with our Creator is to realize that we do fall short of perfection; that this has separated us from Him; and that He loved us so much that He created a way for us to be restored to a personal relationship with Him.

For God so loved the world that he gave his one and only Son, that whoever believes in him shall not perish but have eternal life (John 3:16).

We must turn from or renounce our sinful nature. We must make Jesus Christ our Lord, turning over our wills, our spirits and our bodies for Him to direct. We must rely on the blood sacrifice of Jesus, the innocent God-Man.

He will not force this on anyone: *Here I am! I stand at the door and knock. If anyone hears my voice and opens the door, I will come in and eat with him, and he with me* (Rev. 3:20).

The only thing we have to do to establish this relationship is to seek Him and invite Him into our lives. Then, in obedience, we confess Him to family or friends and are obedient in baptism, worship, prayer and Bible study as we start to mature in this wonderful relationship.

The New Creation

Accepting the Creator through His Son, we realize that we are of far more worth than something that arose through the worthless protoplasm of evolutionary theory. We are a "new creation" (2 Cor. 5:17). We are the "salt of the earth" (Matt. 5:13). We are "the light of the world" (v. 14). We are "children of God" (John 1:12). We are Christ's friends (see 15:14).

Your value and your strength genuinely *soar* when you realize who you are in Christ!

You can easily see that faith in the Designer and trust in His design makes the difference between life and death. If you have not yet accepted the will of this loving Designer for your life, and received His Son as your Savior, won't you simply do it now?

Congratulations! Enjoy!

Notes

Chapter 1

1. George A. Bender, *Great Moments in Medicine* (Detroit: Parke Davis & Company, 1965), pp. 198-207.
2. "AIDS in Heterosexuals," *University of California-Berkeley Wellness Letter* (November 1988): 7.
3. In a community following *kosher* food preparation rules, only certain animals, birds and fish are permissible to eat. According to the Levitical law, animals and birds must be ritually slaughtered by a Jewish person trained in the proper way of killing and preparing the meat. The law of *parve* states that meat and milk dishes should never be eaten or prepared together. This in itself is a sensible health practice because the presence of milk in the stomach inhibits the digestion of meat if they are eaten together. To avoid any chance of contamination of milk and meat products, however, *kosher* kitchens have separate cupboards, dishes, refrigerators and other requirements. *Parve* is an example of how *kosher* laws or "traditions" take a biblical law ("Do not cook a young goat in its mother's milk" [Exod. 23:19; see also 34:26; Deut. 14:21]) and extend that law into a whole subset of extra regulations. It is precisely against this kind of mentality, which legalistically pays more attention to external rules than to the internal condition of a person's heart, that Jesus preached and taught (e.g., Matt. 5-7; Mark 7:1-23).
4. For example, Jesus offended religious Jews by breaking Jewish traditions, intentionally becoming "unclean," by their traditional standards, but without breaking Mosaic law. He ate without washing hands (see Mark 7:3), picked grain and healed on the Sabbath (see Matt. 12:1-12; Mark 2:23-28), didn't fast as did other religious people (see Mark 2:18,19), dined with tax gatherers and sinners (see Luke 5:30), mingled with Gentiles (see 7:1-10), touched and healed lepers and other sick people (see v. 22) and allowed Himself to be touched by sinful women (see v. 39). Ultimately Jesus, the only person ever to have perfectly obeyed God's laws, took the sin of the world upon Himself on the cross, there being made totally defiled for us (see Gal. 3:13; 2 Cor. 5:21; cf. Deut. 21:23). Jesus affirmed the Old Testament law and the prophets in their original prophetic intent, but in Christ the Old Testament laws are completely fulfilled, even though not "one jot nor one tittle" was changed (see Matt. 5:17,18, NKJV).
5. Peter, a very religious Jew and one of Jesus' 12 disciples, had followed Jewish traditions based upon Old Testament dietary restrictions all his life. Peter's vision of the sheet containing "all kinds of four-footed animals of the earth" (Acts 10:14, NKJV)—forbidden ("unclean")—horrified him because he had never eaten anything impure or unclean (see Ezek. 4:14).

   Although many interpret this dream to mean that all things are intended for food, I believe the best interpretation of the vision is that neither the oral traditions nor the law are necessary for salvation. At no time during the vision were the unclean items lowered to the ground so that Peter could eat them. The vision was against the oral tradition of the Jews, saying that they could not eat with nor go into the home of a Gentile. The gospel message was intended for all, including the Gentiles (see Acts 10:38-45; 11:18-21).

   Although Peter seemed to have learned his lesson, the lesson was so radical that later he slipped back into his old legalistic way of thinking. According to Galatians 2:11-14, the apostle Paul remonstrated Peter publicly for hypocrisy because Peter withdrew from the Gentiles and was insisting that they follow Jewish traditions, whereas previously he had eaten with them.
6. On the other hand, Paul would follow the Old Testament ceremonial and dietary laws and Jewish traditions when the salvation of Jewish people was at stake. Paul understood that the Mosaic law has the purpose of leading us to Christ (see Gal. 3:24); it was not necessary for salvation, purification or holiness. However, the law and traditions should be respected by those wanting to win Jewish people to the gospel (see 1 Cor. 9:19,20).
7. J. Macrae, "Nightingale's Spiritual Philosophy and Its Significance for Modern Nursing," *Image*, The Journal of Nursing Scholarship 27:1 (Spring 1995): 8-10.
8. Given the idolatry of the surrounding nations, it is also reasonable to infer (1) that the laws of sexual uncleanness were aimed directly against immoral Canaanite sexual practices (see Lev. 15:2,16,19,25; 18:6,20,22); (2) that the laws concerning dead bodies represented a decisive rejection of all forms of cults of the dead (see Lev. 5:2; Num. 19:14f.); and (3) that animals dedicated to gods other than the one true God—such as the sacred camel of Egypt (see Lev. 11:4); the pig prominent in the Adonis-Tammuz cult (see 11:7); mice, snakes and rabbits (see vv. 6,29-31) that were used in magic; and the dog (see vv. 27,28), sacred to the Phoenicians, Babylonians, Egyptians and Persians—were unclean because of their connection with the worship of foreign gods.
9. Paul emphasized that idolatry was not just sinful, but actually the worship of demons (see 1 Cor. 10:20; cf. Lev. 19:4; Deut. 32:16,17; Ps. 106:37-39; Zech. 13:2). Even foreign lands were unclean because the people worshiped other so-called "gods" in those places (see Amos 7:17). See also Hans-George Link regarding "pure" in the *New International Dictionary of New Testament Theology*, vol. 3, ed. by Colin Brown (Grand Rapids: Zondervan, 1978), pp. 100-108.
10. A clear hygienic purpose is not always or necessarily apparent. For example, a woman is unclean for 7 days after giving birth to a boy, but for 14 days after giving birth to a girl (see Lev. 12:1-5). In some cases, a thing is clean or unclean for no discernible reason other than God said so. (But remember that things that made no sense 200 years ago are now clear with scientific findings.)
11. Sir Robert McGarrison, M.D. and H. M. Sinclair, *Nutrition and Health* (London: Faber and Faber, 1945).
12. F. Gunby, "Battles continue over DES use in fattening cattle," *Journal of American Medical Association* 244(3) (July 1980): 228.
13. Udo Erasmus, *Fats That Kill and Fats that Heal* (Burnaby, B.C., Canada: Alive Books, 1994), p. 253.
14. M. V. Trevivon, "Consumption of Olive Oil, Butter, and Vegetable Oil and Coronary Heart Disease Risk Factors," *Journal of American Medical Association* 263:5 (February 2, 1990): 688-691.

Chapter 2

1. According to this view, some scientists choose to believe in the supernatural, and others do not. The choice itself, to believe or not to believe, has nothing whatever to do with science (which as stated has only to do with the material universe). Rather, the choice is based upon a particular religious worldview: faith, or nonfaith, in a supernatural Creator. The choice to believe in the supernatural is often characterized by those who have chosen not to believe as a choice in favor of superstition and back to the Middle Ages. However, the religious choice for nonbelief is not without its problems.

   Harvard's Nobel prize-winning biologist George Wald, in *Frontiers of Modern Biology on Theories of Origin of Life* (New York: Houghton Mifflin, 1972), p. 187, illustrates this point:

   "There are only two possible explanations as to how life arose: Spontaneous generation arising to evolution or a supernatural creative act of God...There is no other possibility. Spontaneous generation was scientifically disproved 120 years ago by Louis Pasteur and others, but that just leaves us with only one other possibility...that life came as a supernatural act of creation by God, but I can't accept that philosophy because I do not want to believe in God. Therefore I choose to believe in that which I know is scientifically impossible, spontaneous generation leading to evolution."

   Scientists, whether they are physical scientists or social scientists, who do not believe in God, base their unbelief not on science, but on a religious choice to disbelieve in a Creator. Unfortunately, their religious choice to exclude God begs some of the biggest questions that thinking human beings everywhere ask. For example, how did life come about from nonlife? How does personality come from nonpersonality? How can we explain the seemingly perfect design of the eye? Why do humans yearn for justice and beauty? How does nature "decide" anything? Where did all the matter of the universe come from in the first place? When scientists suggest some sort of personality or design in nature, or that matter or life was "spontaneously generated," they are breaking their own rule of limiting the discussion to the material order. They are smuggling in the element of the supernatural and calling it by another name. When scientists speak of spontaneous generation, they are talking outside the boundaries of science; they are talking about God, whether they will admit it or not.

On the other hand, scientists who doggedly refuse to admit God to the realm of acceptable discussion are forced by their presuppositions (their choice not to believe in a supernatural Creator) to put forth the theory of the spontaneous generation of life. They must design theoretical constructs such as macro-evolution to explain the complexity and wonder of life. The very best physical or social scientists can do is to describe data received from the five senses. They can never give an "ought" in any pronouncement without taking off their scientist hats and putting on moral/ethical/religious hats. Ultimately, they must place their full faith in random chance, which leads directly to the belief that we are nothing more than accidents in time, that nothing "out there" cares for us, and that we are nothing more than a complex primal ooze.

2. See George Marsden, *The Soul of the American University: From Protestant Establishment to Establishment of Nonbelief* (New York: Oxford University Press, 1994), especially pp. 113-122.

3. S. I. McMillen, *None of These Diseases* (Grand Rapids: Fleming Revell Co., 1979).

4. M. A. Ruffer, "Studies in Paleopathology in Egypt," *Journal of Pathology and Bacteriology* 18 (1913): 149-62; P. E. Ross, "Eloquent Remains," *Scientific American* 266:5 (May 1992): 114-19; C. T. Marx, "Examination of Eleven Egyptian Mummies," *RasioGraphics* 6:2 (March 1986): 321-325.

5. *Vital Statistics of the United States, 1991*, cited in the *Cancer Journal for Clinicians* 41:1 (February 1991): 22.

6. B. F. Feingold, "Dietary Management of Behavior and Learning Disabilities," *Nutrition and Behavior* (Philadelphia: Miller Publishing Co., 1981), p. 76.

7. G. A. Burkhart, "Aspirin and Colorectal Cancer," *Annals of Internal Medicine* 123:5 (September 1, 1995): 390-391.

8. *Vital Statistics of the United States, 1991*, cited in the *Cancer Journal for Clinicians* 41:1 (February 1991): 10.

9. J. H. Weisburger, Ph.D. and E. L. Wynder, M.D., "Nutrition and Cancer—A Review of Relevant Mechnanisms," *The Cancer Bulletin* 34:4 (1982): 128-135.

10. E. Cheraskin, M.D., William M. Ringsdorf, M.D., and J. W. Clark, D.D.S., *Diet and Disease* (New Canaan, Conn.: Keats Publishing, 1968), p. 308.

11. J. W. Anderson, "Plant Fiber: Carbohydrate and Lipid Metabolism," *American Journal of Clinical Nutrition* 32:2 (February 1979): 346-363.

12. Michail Wargovich, M.D., *The Cancer Bulletin* 376:1 (1985): 3-4.

13. H. King, "Diabetes in Adults Is Now a Third World Problem," *Ethnicity and Disease,* Supplement S, World Health Organization (1993): 67-74.

14. R. Williams, "Epidemiological and Geographic Factors in Diabetes," *Eye* 7:2 (1993): 202-204.

15. Anderson, ibid.

16. Guy. R. Newell, M.D., series ed., "Cancer Prevention: Update for Physicians," *The Cancer Bulletin* 37:2 (1985): 91-93.

17. J. D. Beasley, *Food for Recovery* (New York: Crown Trade Paperbacks, 1994), p. 42.

18. William Philpott, M.D., *Brain Allergies* (New Canaan, Conn.: Keats Publications, 1980), pp. 15-18, 90-109.

19. Personal communications with the camp director, Lester Roloff, in Corpus Christi, Texas.

20. Lendon Smith, M.D., *Feed Your Kids Right* (Jackson, Tenn.: Professional Books, 1979).

21. K. Ward and J. Anderson, "High-carbohydrate, High-fiber Diets for Insulin-treated Men with Diabetes Mellitus," *American Journal of Clinical Nutrition* 32:11 (November 1979): 2312-2321.

22. Nathan Pritikin, *Live Longer Now* (New York: Grosset & Dunlap, 1974).

Chapter 3

1. "The Food Insects Newsletter" (May 1995): 1.

2. "Harmful Fish," *World Book Encyclopedia,* vol. 9 (Chicago: Field Enterprises, 1979), p. 141.

3. Ethyl Nelson, M.D., "The Eden Diet and Modern Nutritional Research" (proceedings of the 1992 Twin Cities Creation Conference in Minneapolis, Minn.), pp. 57-60.

4. Ibid., p. 59.

5. Ibid., p. 58.

6. D. Burkitt, "Varicose Veins Among the Masai?" *Lancet* 1:808 (April 1973): 890.

7. G. B. Walker, A.R.P., D. P. Burkitt and N. S. Pointor, "Dietary fiber and disease," *JAMA* 229 (1973): 1068-1074.

8. Cited by J. White in *The Study of the Intelligent Design of the Universe* (Branson, Mo.: Creation Science, n.d.), p. 5.

Chapter 4

1. Notice that in the same chapter God condemns unholy sexual relations and eating unclean meats (see Rom. 14:1-23; 1 Cor. 8:8; Col. 2:16; 1 Tim. 4:4; Heb. 9:10; 13:9). Obviously, for the Israelites these forbidden items had both moral and hygienic applications. For Christians, however, there is no spiritual defilement in eating unclean meats. On the other hand, we can afford to ask, is the consumption of unclean meats wise? Is it hygienic? Read on.

2. H. M. Morris, Ph.D., *Pre Genesis Record* (San Diego, Calif.: Institute of Creation Research, 1976), pp. 242-262.

3. Jonathan Henry, Ph.D., "Fate of the Ethnic Groups in the Table of Nations" (a paper presented at 1992 Twin Cities Creation Conference in Minneapolis, Minn.), p. 91.

4. P. K. Lewin, "Possible Origin of Human Aids," *Canadian Medical Association Journal* 132 (1985): 1110.

5. R. C. Gallo, "Antibodies to Simian T-Lymphotropic Retrovirus Type III in African Green Monkeys and Recognition of STLV-III Viral Proteins by AIDS and Related Sera," *Lancet* 8 (June 1985): 1330-1332.

6. J. I. Slaff and J. K. Brubaker, *The Aids Epidemic* (New York: Warner Books, 1985), p. 112.

7. C. Y. Chuang, "Aids in the Republic of China, 1992," *Clinical Infectious Diseases* 17:Suppl. 2 (November 1993): 5337-5340.

8. C. Bun, "Homosexuality and Biology," *Atlantic Monthly* 271:3 (March 1993): 47-65.

9. Virginia H. Masters and William Johnson, *Homosexuality in Perspective* (Boston: Little, Brown, 1979).

10. Joe McIlhaney, Jr., M.D., ed., "Condoms Ineffective Against Human Papilloma Virus," *Sexual Health Update* 2:2 (April 1994): 1-2.

11. "Condoms Won't Prevent Transmission of Human Papillomavirus," *Family Planning News* 22:1 (June 1992): 1.

12. H. M. Bauer, "Genital Human Papillomavirus Infection in Female University Students as Determined by a PcR-Based Method," *Journal of the American Medical Association* 265:4 (1991): 472-475.

13. Susan Weller, "A Meta-Analysis of Condom Effectiveness in Reducing Sexually Transmitted HIV," *Social Science and Medicine* 36:12 (June 1993): 1635-1644.

14. J. P. Zhang, "An Epidemiology Study on HIV Infection in Ruili County Yunnan Province," *Chinese Journal of Epidemiology* 12:1 (February 1991): 9-11.

15. "Heterosexual Spread," *Mortality and Morbidity Weekly Report,* 34 (September 20, 1985): 561-563.

16. Susan Weller, "A Meta-Analysis of Condom Effectiveness in Reducing Sexually Transmitted HIV," *Social Science and Medicine* 36:12 (June 1993): 1735-1644.

17. Lorraine Day, M.D., *AIDS* (Rockport, Mass.: Rockport Press, 1991).

18. N. Wang, "First Reported Case of Aids in China," *Chinese Medical Journal* 71:12 (December 1991): 671-673.

19. G. T. Stewart, "Life-styles Plus HIV Equal Death," *Genetica* 95:1-3 (1995): 173-193.

20. Arno Karlen, *Man and Microbes* (New York: G. P. Putman's Sons, 1995), p. 66.

Chapter 5

1. Albert Anderson, M.D., "Creation Health—Forgotten Medical Science," *Medical Imaging* 17:21 (1978): 20.

2. George Thampy, Ph.D., "Effect of Fasting and Lacto-vegetarian Diet on Glucose Tolerance and Weightless Maintenance in Obese and Obese Type II Diabetics." Paper presented at conference "Food Intake and Body Weight Regulations" (2252), *Medical Training Institute Newsletter* (June 1992): 2.

3. J. Kjeldsen-Kragh, M.D., "Controlled Trial of Fasting and One-year Vegetarian Diet in Rheumatic Arthritis," *Lancet* 338:8772 (October 12, 1991): 899-902.

4. Yuri Nikolayave and Allan Cott, "Continued Fasting Treatment of Schizophrenics in the U.S.S.R.," *Schizophrenia* 1 (1969): 44.

5. Allan Cott, M.D., "Treating Schizophrenic Children," *Schizophrenia* 1 (1967): 3.

6. William Philpott, M.D., *Brain Allergies* (New Canaan, Conn.: Keats Publishing, 1980), p. 28.

7. Karolyn Gazella, "Addictions: Breaking Free Is Possible," *Health Counselor* 7:1 (1995): 27-31.

8. Joseph Beasley, M.D. and J. M. A. Swift, *The Kellogg Report* (Bard College Center, N.Y.: Institute of Health Policy and Practice, 1989), p. 371.

9. Joseph Beasley, M.D., *Food for Recovery* (New York: Crown Trade Paperbacks, 1994), p. 5.

10. Richard Weindruch, M.D., "Dietary Restriction in Mice," *Science* 215:4538 (March 12, 1982): 1415-1418.

11. "How to Discover the Rewards of Fasting," *Basic Care Bulletin* 4. Medical Training Institute of America, Box 3113, Oak Brook, IL 60522-3113.

Chapter 6

1. P. Vijayagopalan, "Effect of Dietary Starches on the Serum, Aorta, and Hepatic Levels in Cholesterol-fed Rats," *Atherosclerosis* 11:2 (March-April 1970): 257-264.

2. David Green, *Molecular Insights into the Living Process* (New York: Academic Press, 1967), pp. 406-407.

3. Robert Jastrow, *Until the Sun Dies* (New York: W. W. Norton, 1977), p. 17.

4. William M. Curtis III, "The Origin of Diverse Languages and Races" (proceedings of the Twin Cities Creation Conference in Minneapolis, Minn.), p. 178; P. R. S. Mooney, *Ur of the*

Chaldees (Ithaca, N.Y.: Cornell University Press, 1982); Holger Pederson, *The Discovery of Language* (Bloomington, Ind.: Indiana University Press, 1962); Merritt Ruhlen, *A Guide to the World's Languages*, Vol. I (Palo Alto, Calif.: Stanford University Press, 1987).

5. Mary Ruth Swope and D. A. Darbro, *Green Leaves of Barley* (Phoenix: Swope Enterprises, Inc., 1983).

6. "Nutrition News," *Prevention* (September 1995): 65.

7. Nicholas Freydberg, *The Food Additives Book* (New York: Bantam Books, 1982), pp. 572-576.

8. Udo Erasmus, *Fats that Heal, Fats that Kill* (Burnaby, B.C., Canada: Alive Books, 1994), pp. 93-98.

9. Adelle Davis, *Let's Eat Right* (New York: Harcourt Brace & Co., 1970), p. 63.

10. Sheldon Margen, M.D., *The Wellness Encyclopedia of Food and Nutrition* (Berkeley: The University of California at Berkeley, 1992), p. 348.

Chapter 7

1. Marie Krause and Kathleen Mahan, *Food, Nutrition and Diet Therapy* (West Washington Square, Pa.: W. B. Saunders, 1979), p. 55.

2. Petr Skrabanek, *The Death of Humane Medicine* (Trinity College, Ireland: Social Affairs Unit, 1995). Reviewed by Dr. Petr Skrabanek in *National Review* (May 1, 1995): 43-47.

3. Ibid.

4. Mary Enig, "More on Coronary Heart Disease: Sense and Nonsense," *New England Journal of Medicine* 331(9) (September 1, 1994): 615.

5. Michael DeBakey, "Correlation Between Blood Cholesterol and Atherosclerosis," *Journal of American Medical Association* 189 (1964): 655-659.

6. Skrabanek, loc. cit.

7. Udo Erasmus, *Fats That Heal, Fats That Kill* (Burnaby, B.C., Canada: Alive Books, 1994), pp. 6-8.

8. Ibid.

9. Ibid., p. 4.

10. Enig, loc. cit.

11. Beatrice Hunter, *Natural Food and Farming* 40:2 (March 1994): 34.

12. Francisco Perez, M.D., "The Beneficial Effects of Olive Oil on Health," (Olive Oil Seminar, Cordoba, Spain, January 21, 1993).

13. Surgeon General's Report, Washington, D.C., Publication No. 88-50210, 1988, Department of Health and Human Services.

14. Ronald Mensink and Martin Katan, "Dietary Oils, Serum Lipoproteins and Coronary Heart Disease," *American Journal of Clinical Nutrition* 61:Suppl. 6 (June 1995): 13685-13735.

15. Erasmus, loc. cit.

Chapter 8

1. Jim Martin, Th.D., tour director for Hebrew University. Two-week lecture series attended 1993.

2. Phil Gunby, "It's Not Fishy: Fruit of the Sea May Foil Cardiovascular Disease," *Journal of the American Medical Association* 247:8 (February 12, 1982): 729-782.

3. Udo Erasmus, *Fats That Heal, Fats That Kill* (Burnaby, B.C., Canada: Alive Books, 1994), pp. 43, 73.

4. Priscilla Briney, "Longhorn Lite—A Colorado Trademark," *The Longhorn Scene* (July/August 1986): 28.

5. Erasmus, op. cit. p. 225.

6. Ibid., p. 275.

7. Ibid., p. 309.

8. M. Krause, *Food, Nutrition and Diet Therapy* (Philadelphia: W. B. Sanders Co., 1979), p. 70.

9. *University of California Berkeley Wellness Letter* (February 1986): 3.

10. Erasmus, op. cit. p. 219.

11. Ibid., pp. 225-226.

12. Ibid., pp. 232-233.

13. E. Mindell, *Unsafe at Any Meal* (New York: Warner Books, 1987), P. 131.

14. R. Saynor, "Effect of a Marine Oil High in Eicosapentaenoic Acid on Blood Lipids and Coagulation," *Therapeutic Hematology and Nutrition* 8 (1980): 378-379.

15. David Macht, M.D., "An Experimental Pharmacological Appreciation of Leviticus XI and Deuteronomy XIV," *Bulletin of Historical Medicine*, Johns Hopkins University, 47:1 (April 1953): 444-450.

16. A. Marinculic, D. Rapic, J. Brglez, N. Dzakula and D. Stojiljkovic, "Epidemiological Survey of Trichinellosis in Yugoslavia," *Southeast Asian Journal of Tropical Medicine & Public Health* 22:Suppl. (December 1991): 302-307.

17. Jane Cahill and Peter Warnock, "It Had to Happen, Scientist Examines Ancient Bathrooms of Romans 586 B.C." *BAR* (May/June 1991): 64-49.

18. J. Bjorland, D. Brown, H. R. Gamble and J. B. McAuley, "Trichinella Spiralis Infection in Pigs in the Bolivian Altiplano," *Veterinary Parasitology* 47:3-4 (May 1993): 349-354.

19. D. G. Baker, J. D. Bryant, J. F. Urban Jr. and J. K. Lunney, "Swine Immunity to Selected Parasites," *Veterinary Immunology and Immunopathology* 43:1-3 (October 1994): 127-133.

20. W. J. Zimmermann, J. H. Steele and I. G. Kagan, "Trichiniasis in the U.S. Population, 1966-70: Prevalence and Epidemiologic Factors," *Health Services Reports* 88:7 (August-September 1973): 606-623.

21. T. Yamaguchi, "Present Status of Trichinellosis in Japan" (Review), *Southeast Asian Journal of Tropical Medicine and Public Health* 22:Suppl. (December 1991): 295-301.

22. A. Marinculic, D. Rapic, J. Brglez, N. Dzakula and D. Stojiljkovic, "Epidemiological Survey of Trichinellosis in Yugoslavia," *Southeast Asian Journal of Tropical Medicine and Public Health* 22:Suppl. (December 1991): 302-307.

23. Chriastoph Scholtissek, M.D., "Cultivating a Killer Virus," *National History* (January 1992): 2.

24. "Keeping Livestock Healthy," *1942 Yearbook of Agriculture*, (Washington: United States Government Printing Office, 1942), pp. 673-828.

25. S. R. Ripped, "Infectious Diseases Associated with Moleskin Shellfish Consumption," *Clinical Microbiology Reviews* 7:4 (October 1994): 419-25. See also J. Eastaugh, "Infectious and Toxic Syndromes from Fish and Shellfish Consumption," *Archives of Internal Medicine* 150:3 (March 1990): 683.

26. J. Pekkanen, "Is your Seafood Safe?" *Reader's Digest* (July 1995): 122.

27. M. D. Hunt, W. E. Woodward, B. H. Keswick and H. L. Dupont, "Seroepidemiology of Cholera in Gulf Coastal Texas," *Applied and Environmental Microbiology* 54:7 (July 1988): 1673-1677.

28. P. H. Rheinstein, M.S., and K. C. Klontz, M.D., "Shellfish-borne Illnesses," *American Family Physician*, U.S. Drug Food and Drug Administration (June 1993): 1837.

29. K. Clark, Ph.D. and D.V.M., Director of Texas Health Department. Quoted in *Organic Gardening* (April 1995): 10.

30. L. Frumkin, M. D. and J. Leonard, M.D., *Questions and Answers on AIDS* (Los Angeles: PMICF, 1994).

31. Source: I. Doucet, "Desert Storm Syndrome: Sick Soldiers and Dead Children," *Medicine and War* 10(3) (July-September 1994): 183-194.

32. D. P. Hajjar, K. B. Pomerantz, D. J. Falcone, B. B. Weksler and A. J. Grant, "Herpes Simplex Virus Infection in Human Arterial Cells: Implications in Arteriosclerosis," *Journal of Clinical Investigation* 80:5 (November 1987): 1317-1321.

33. A. Dalsgaard, O. Serichantalergs, T. Shimada, O. Sethabutr and P. Echeverria, "Prevalence of Vibrio Cholera with Heat-stable Enterotoxin," *Journal of Medical Microbiology* 43:3 (September 1995): 216-220.

34. J. W. Chambers, "An Outbreak of Viral Gastroenteritis Associated with Adequately Prepared Oysters," *Epidemiology and Infection* 115:1(January 1995): 163-167.

35. *Consumer Reports* (February 1992): 112.

36. L. Skoldstam and K. E. Magnusson, "Fasting, Intestinal Permeability, and Rheumatoid Arthritis," *Rheumatic Diseases Clinics of North America* 17:2 (May 1991): 363-371.

37. J. Kjeldsen-Kragh, M. Haugen, C. F. Borchgrevink, E. Laerum, E. M. Mowinkel, K. Hovi and O. Forre, "Controlled Trial of Fasting and One-year Vegetarian Diet in Rheumatoid Arthritis," *Lancet* 338:8772 (October 12, 1991): 899-902.

38. H. P. Rhomberg, "Excessive egg consumption and hypercholesterol anemia," *British Medical Journal* 1(6019) (1976 May 15): 1188-1189.

39. M. Flynn, "Serum Lipids and Eggs," *Journal of the American Dietetic Association* 86:11 (November 1986): 1541-1542.

40. "Egg on the Face of Old Research?" *Minneapolis Star Tribune* (November 19, 1995).

41. Wm. Douglas, M.D., *The Milk of Human Kindness* (Lakemont, Ga.: Copple House Books, Inc., 1985), p. 213.

Chapter 9

1. B. Hirschel, "Dr. Atkins dietetic revolution: a critique," *Journal of Swiss Medicine* 107(29) (July 23, 1977): 1017-1025.

2. Nathan Pritikin, *Live Longer Now* (New York: Grosset & Dunlap Publishers, 1974), p. X111.

3. Rudolph Ballentine, M.D., *Diet and Nutrition* (Homesdale, Pa.: The Himalayan International Institute, 1978), p. 62; Cecil Tonsley, *Honey for Health* (New York: Award Books, 1979); Joe M. Parkhill, *Honey* (Lenexa, Kans.: Cookbook Publishers, 1979).

4. Medical Training Institute of America, *Basic Care Bulletin*, no. 4, pp. 16-18.

5. Ballentine, *Diet and Nutrition*, p. 62.

6. Joe Nichols, M.D., *Please Doctor, Do Something* (Joe Nichols, 1972). Dr. Nichols is the ex-president of the Natural Foods Association.

7. Sheldon Margen, M.D. *The Wellness Encyclopedia of Food and Nutrition* (New York: Rebus Health Letter Associates, 1992), p. 326.

8. Consumer Safety Network, P.O. Box 789634, Dallas, TX 75378.

9. Earl Mindell, *Unsafe at Any Meal* (New York: Warner Books, 1987).

10. The American Institute for Cancer Research, *Diet, Nutrition, and Cancer* (Washington, D.C.: National Academy Press, 1982), p. 310.

11. *University of California-Berkeley Wellness Letter* (August 1, 1988): 1.

12. William Dufty, *Sugar Blues* (New York: Warner Books, 1975).

13. John Yudkin, M.D., *Sweet and Dangerous* (New York: Bantam Books, 1971), p. 98.

14. Joe M. Parkhill, *Honey, God's Gift for Health and Beauty* (Lenexa, Kans.: Cookbook Publisher, 1979).

Chapter 10

1. J. O. Hill, H. Douglas and J. C. Peters, "Obesity Treatment: Can Diet Composition Play a Role?" *Annals of Internal Medicine* 119(2):7 (1993): 694-697.
2. *The Doctors Book of Home Remedies,* by the editors of *Prevention* magazine (Emmaus, Pa.: Bantum Books-Rodale Press, 1990).
3. B. J. Hunter, "Prospective Study of the Intake of Vitamin C, E, and A and the Risk of Breast Cancer," *New England Journal of Medicine* 329:4 (February 1993): 234.
4. R. Greenberg, M.D., "A Clinical Trial of Antioxident Vitamins to Prevent Colorectal Adenoma," *New England Journal of Medicine* 221:3 (July 21, 1994): 141.
5. Anonymous, "Position of the American Dietetic Association: Phytochemicals and Functional Foods," *Journal of the American Dietetics Association* (April 1995): 493-496.
6. Earl Mindell, *Unsafe at Any Meal* (New York: Warner Books, 1987), pp. 37-41.
7. "Morbidity and Mortality Weekly Report," *New England Journal of Medicine* 35(16) (April 25, 1986): 254-258.
8. James Marshall, Ph.D. "Eat Well," *Family Circle* 23 (June 1992): 62.
9. Mindell, op. cit., 21.
10. *Univesity of California-Berkeley Wellness Letter* 5:10 (July 1989): 1.

Chapter 11

1. J. Lyon, "Herbal Arsenal," *Chicago Tribune* (Sunday, December 20, 1992): 11.
2. David Darom, Ph.D., *Beautiful Plants of the Bible* (Herzlfia, Israel: Palphot, Ltd., n.d.).
3. James R. Balch, M.D. and A. Phyllis Balch, C.N.C., *Prescription for Nutritional Healing* (Garden City, N.Y.: Avery Publishing, 1990), p. 47.
4. Darom, op. cit., p. 8.
5. Eddie Palmer, M.D., personal communications to my class at Baylor College of Medicine, Houston, Tex., 1965.
6. N. Marioka, *Cancer Immunology* 37(5) (October 1993): 316-322.
7. A. P. McEchoy, *Avian Disease* 38(2) (April-June 1994): 329-333.
8. Lazzeri, *Scandinavian Journal of Urology* 28(4) (December 1994): 409-412.
9. Mary Ruth Swope, *Green Leaves of Barley* (Phoenix: Swope Enterprises, 1987).
10. Balch and Balch, op. cit., p. 46.

Chapter 12

1. National Resources Defense Council, *Rural Arkansas* (October 1995): 4.
2. Ibid.
3. Joseph M. Price, M.D., *Coronaries/Cholesterol/Chlorine* (New York: Berkeley Publishing Group, 1981).
4. "Fluoridation Facts: Answers to Questions About Fluoridation" pamphlet, American Dental Association, 211 E. Chicago Ave., Chicago, IL 60611.
5. "The Use of Fluoride-containing Toothpastes in Young Children: The Scientific Evidence for Recommending a Small Quantity," *Pediatric Dentistry* 14:6 (November-December 1992): 384-387; L. Wm. Greenberg, "Excessive Fluoride," op. cit., 16:5 (September-November 1994): 335.

6. P. A. Palma and E. W. Adcock III, "Human Milk and Breast-feeding," *Practical Therapeutics* 24 (1981): 173-181.
7. P. A. Newcomb, "Lactation and a Reduced Risk of Premenopausal Breast Cancer," *New England Journal of Medicine* 330:2 (1994): 81.
8. William Campbell Douglass, M.D., *The Milk of Human Kindness Is Not Pasteurized* (Lakemont, Ga.: Copple House Books, Inc., 1986).
9. J. Gregory, "Denaturation of the Folacin-binding Protein in Pasteurized Milk Products," *Journal of Nutrition* 112:7 (July 1982): 1329-1338.
10. J. M. Farber, "Thermal Resistance of Listeria Monocytogenes in Inoculated and Naturally Contaminated Raw Milk," *International Journal of Food Microbiology* 7:4 (December 1988): 277-286.
11. E. V. McCollum, "Getting the Most out of Milk," *Journal of Nutrition* 91:2, Suppl. 1:6-11 (February 1967).
12. K. A. Oster, *The American Journal of Medicine* 290:6 (April 18, 1974): 913.
13. S. Yanagi, "Comparative Effects of Milk, Yogurt, Butter and Margarine on Mammary Tumorigensis," *Cancer Detection and Prevention* 18:6 (1994): 415-420.
14. Kathleen Baldinger, *The World's Oldest Health Plan* (New York: Starburst, 1994), p. 12.
15. B. L. Banstra's article about "wine" in *The International Standard Bible Encyclopedia,* vol. 4 (Grand Rapids: Wm. B. Eerdmans Publishing Co.: 1979), p. 1070.
16. A. P. Thomas, "Effects of Ethanol on the Contractile Function of the Heart," *Alcoholism, Clinical and Experimental Research* 18:1, pp. 121-131.
17. S. Ahlawat, "Effects of ethyl alcohol on coronary circulation in patients with angina," *The International Journal of Cardiology* 33(3) (December 1991): 385-391.
18. C. Tabin, "The Initiation of the Limb Bud: Growth Factors," *Cell* 80:5 (March 10, 1995): 671-674; S. B. Siwach, "Alcohol and coronary artery disease," *The International Journal of Cardiology* 44(2) (1994): 157-162.
19. J. Jowsey, "Osteoporosis," *Postgraduate Medicine* 60 (1976): 75-79.
20. R. D. Lindeman, *Magnesium in Health and Disease* (Deerfield, Ill.: SP Medical and Scientific Books, 1980), pp. 236-245.

Appendix 1

1. R. B. Sheddelle, M.D., "Type-A Behavior Found Not Linked to Heart Disease," *Medical World News* (March 28, 1983): 23-27.
2. Dean Ornish, M.D., *Dr. Dean Ornish's Program for Reversing Heart Disease Without Surgery or Drugs* (New York: Ballantine Books, 1992), p. 86.
3. R. P. Mensink, "Effect of Dietary Cis and Trans Fatty Acids on Serum Lipoprotein Levels in Humans," *Journal of Lipid Research* 33:10 (October 1992): 1493-1501.
4. Kenneth R. Pelletier, *Mind as Healer Mind as Slayer* (New York: Dell Publishing, Co., 1977), p. 110.

Appendix 2

1. J. B. Hudson and G. H. Towers, "Therapeutic Potential of Plan Photosensitizers," *Pharmacology and Therapeutics* 49:3 (1991): 181-222.
2. Charles Darwin, *Origin of Species* (London: J. M. Dent & Sons, 1971), p. 167.
3. J. L. Tennant, M.D., "How to Keep from Going Blind," (Duncanville, Tex.: Dallas Eye Institute, n.d.), pp. 2-4.
4. "Not Equal Under the Sun," *University of California-Berkeley Wellness Letter* 4:11 (August 1988): 7.
5. E. Cheraskin, M.D. and W. M. Ringsdorf Jr., *Psychodietetics* (Briarcliff Manor, N.Y.: Stein and Day, 1974), pp. 141-42.
6. Ibid., p. 14.
7. I. J. Deary, "Hostile Personality and Risks of Arterial Disease in the General Population," *Psychosomatic Medicine* 56:3 (May/June 1994): 197-202.
8. E. C. Suariz, E. Harlan, E. Peoples and R. B. Williams Jr., "Cardiovascular and Emotional Responses in Women: The Role of Hostility and Harassment," *Health and Psychology* 12:6 (November 1993): 459-468.
9. K. Eliasson, "A Dietary Fiber Supplement in the Treatment of Mild Hypertension: A Randomized, Double-blind, Placebo-controlled Trial," *Journal of Hypertension* 2 (February 1992): 195-199.
10. M. Haugen, "Changes in Laboratory Variables in Rheumatoid Arthritis Patients During a Trial of Fasting and One-year Vegetarian Diet," *Scandinavian Journal of Rheumatology* 24:2 (1995): 85-93.

Index

Date Due

Code 4386-04, CLS-4, Broadman Supplies, Nashville, Tenn., Printed in U.S.A.